# THE BRITISH ARMY CHALLENGE BOOK

# THE BRITISH ARMY CHALLENGE BOOK

### Over 100 Brain Teasers, Mind Games, Puzzles and Challenges to Test Your Limits!

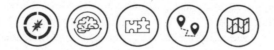

## DR GARETH MOORE

HarperCollins*Publishers*

The puzzles in this book are based on the kind of challenges that you might face in certain situations in the British Army. The puzzles are designed to help train your mind, and should not be treated as actual tests to enter the British Army. Any activities or operations described in the text have been devised purely for the purposes of the puzzles in this book, to provide some practical context, and in no way document real activities. The military activities in this book should only be carried out by professionals in the British Army.

HarperCollins*Publishers*
1 London Bridge Street
London SE1 9GF
www.harpercollins.co.uk

HarperCollinsPublishers
1st Floor, Watemarque Building, Ringsend Road
Dublin 4, Ireland

First published by HarperCollins*Publishers* 2019

5 7 9 10 8 6 4

Dr Gareth Moore asserts the moral right to be
identified as the author of this work

All illustrations courtesy of the author, with the following
exceptions: pp ii, 1, 9, 10, 12 (compass, *also* pp 35, 188, 274), 16,
18, 19, 20, 21, 37, 49, 97, 123 (tyres), 131, 144 (Morse code),
146, 147, 164, 165, 170, 171, 172, 183, 195, 217, 221
(sun and figure), 222 (sun), 225 @Shutterstock.com

Logo on p vii supplied by the British Army

British Army logos are trademarks of the UK Secretary of
State for Defence and used under licence

A catalogue record of this book is available from the British Library

ISBN 978-0-00-835685-9

Printed and Bound in the UK using 100% Renewable Electricity at
CPI Group (UK) Ltd

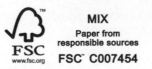

MIX
Paper from
responsible sources
FSC™ C007454

This book is produced from independently certified FSC™
paper to ensure responsible forest management.
For more information visit: www.harpercollins.co.uk/green

# CONTENTS

# FOREWORD

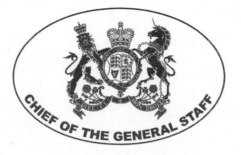

Life is all about finding solutions to today's pressing problems, in an age where increasing complexity, competition and exponential change surround us all. Nowhere is that more important than in the British Army, where problem-solving is an essential skill.

To be the best Army that we can be, we need people who can think clearly and logically, and who enjoy solving puzzles.

So I hope you enjoy this collection of military-based problems and that they sharpen your own problem-solving skills. If you want to take these challenges to the next level, then we are always looking for bright young men and women to join the team. Have fun!

*Mark Carleton-Smith*

General Sir Mark Carleton-Smith KCB CBE ADC Gen
Chief of the General Staff

# INTRODUCTION

The puzzles in this book cover a wide range of skills that a member of the British Army might be expected to have. Of course, the army is all about teamwork, and different people have different specialities, so naturally you will find some puzzles easier than others, depending on your own experience and abilities.

The first chapter, 'In the Field', covers the types of skills you might need in the field, such as making sense of maps, observing important details in landscapes or making quick deductions from limited information.

Being in the British Army requires you to continually adapt and learn new skills, so in the 'Cognitive Testing' chapter you will start with a puzzle familiar to most people – a standard sudoku – and then work through three separate 'obstacle courses' that will give you a thorough test of your cognitive skills. Only the very best will manage to solve every puzzle, however, so if you become completely stuck on a puzzle then it's okay to move on to the next one. You can always go back to it later, once you have more experience.

For the 'Teamwork' chapter, you'll need someone to help you out, since these puzzles are all about solving challenges as a team. Four or more is a good number to have in a team, but most tasks can be completed with just two if necessary. Some tasks require physical props, but you can substitute alternatives if you don't have easy access to the required objects. And if some challenges aren't practical in your current location then skip over them and save them for another day.

The 'Survival' chapter contains a range of puzzles that will test a wide variety of skills, including your code-breaking aptitude, your ability to think logically and quickly, your memory and even your general knowledge.

Finally, in the 'Case Study' chapter you will have a chance to challenge yourself with a full-on British Army-training scenario. It will be up to you to take in all the information and parameters of the situation, and devise a full plan for all the people involved. You'll then have a chance to read through a detailed discussion on how you might have tackled it, to see how your choices compared.

# CHAPTER 1

# [ IN THE FIELD ]

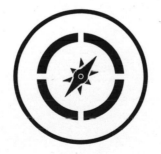

# FIELDCRAFT

Fieldcraft is the collective name for the tactical techniques used by soldiers to survive and operate in close proximity with the enemy. It encapsulates the methods of movement, camouflage and self-discipline necessary for soldiers to remain unseen and undetected on the battlefield.

Until the nineteenth century, soldiers dressed in brightly coloured uniforms. These colours were necessary so that commanders could identify their troops on a smoke-shrouded battlefield. Although this emphasis on visibility might seem misguided to modern eyes, in an era dominated by inaccurate gunpowder weapons and before radio communications, bright uniforms allowed soldiers to be manoeuvred in large formations, often shoulder to shoulder.

The battlefield became an increasingly lethal place as the effects of the Industrial Revolution were felt. Smokeless propellants, precision-engineered artillery, rifled small arms and automatic machine guns combined to make the concentration of troops impossible. Instead, armies began to disperse in order to dilute the effects of industrialisation; they adopted dull-coloured uniforms, which allowed soldiers to blend into the environment in which they operated, and they adopted techniques like entrenching to both protect themselves and deceive the enemy.

Later still, from the Second World War onwards, technology such as night vision, infrared and thermal-imaging equipment allowed adversaries to see each other at all times and in all weathers. Survival on the battlefield became more difficult without effective camouflage, both from view, by the use of specially patterned materials, and from other methods of detection, by thermal and infrared protections. As virtually any movement brought the risk of becoming a target, soldiers learned methods of movement that maximised the chances of remaining unseen by the enemy, using even the smallest advantage offered by the landscape to remain obscured.

These skills, which developed from the late-Victorian era onwards in reaction to an increasingly deadly battlefield, are the cornerstones of modern fieldcraft and are critical to a soldier's ability to survive in that most dangerous of environments. They must be practised continually – until they become almost autonomic – and tested regularly in simulated battle scenarios. The operating environment does not, however, stand still and neither do the techniques of fieldcraft. The modern battlefield is dominated by equipment that can see and target even the slightest surface movement: intelligence-gathering equipment, drones and satellite-enabled precision targeting are just the latest technologies to challenge soldiers' survivability.

What, then, is the future of fieldcraft? Fundamentally, the tactics, techniques and procedures practised by today's soldiers remain both their most effective protection and the only way to engage the enemy in battle and win. It must be borne in mind, however, that the battlefield is continually evolving: deception, disguise and digging will characterise future conflict, as soldiers attempt to avoid enemy surveillance and targeting. Tomorrow's army will continue to practise skills learned from the wars of the past, but it will adapt and innovate to be ready to fight the wars of the future.

# LOGICAL REASONING

You may not always have a complete set of information, yet you will be able to infer everything you need to know from the information you *do* have.

In each of the following five situations, you are given a limited amount of information and must work out the remainder of what you need to know by logical deduction.

## 1. ANTI-POACHING

You are a second lieutenant in charge of a unit of six soldiers, who have been deployed in Malawi to help combat poachers.

You have split the unit into three pairs of soldiers and assigned each pair a colour: green, red or blue. Each pair is helping to protect a different animal from poachers: leopards, elephants or rhinoceroses.

Using the following clues, can you work out which soldiers are in which pair, and which animal they are looking after?

The soldiers' names are Michael, Priti, Rita, Jess, Liam and Elijah.

- The green pair is protecting rhinoceroses
- Rita is not looking after elephants, and is not in the same pair as Jess
- Elijah and Priti are in the same pair
- Liam is helping to guard leopards from poaching
- Jess is in the blue pair
- Michael is not in the pair protecting rhinoceroses

Assign each soldier to a pair in the table below, and identify the animal they are guarding:

|  | Green pair | Red pair | Blue pair |
|---|---|---|---|
| **Soldiers** |  |  |  |
| **Animal** |  |  |  |

## 2. FEEDING THE TROOPS

You are an army chef in charge of feeding 300 soldiers. You plan nutritious dinners, and also eat them yourself. On Monday, Tuesday and Wednesday this week you had a different meal each day, accompanying each with a different drink.

Using the following clues, can you work out what you ate and drank at dinner each day?

- The drinks you chose were coffee, tea and water, and the meals were lasagne, chicken tikka and Irish stew
- You had lasagne the day before the Irish stew
- You drank tea with your meal on Wednesday
- The day you had chicken tikka, you drank water
- You had the dinner with water earlier in the week than the one with coffee

## 3. ARMY PROTECTED PATROL VEHICLES

Your unit has been assigned the task of transporting troops on a patrol mission in the field, and you need to choose the best vehicle for your mission. The British Army has a selection of versatile patrol vehicles that can be used in combat, offering protection from landmines and other threats.

You have narrowed the choice down to three: the Ridgback, the Foxhound and the Panther. You know that the vehicle needs to be able to travel at 70 mph and carry at least four soldiers. Using the statements below, work out the speed and crew capacity of each vehicle, and therefore which one is the best for the job.

- The Panther can carry one more person than the Ridgback
- The Foxhound is 20 mph faster than the Panther
- The Ridgback is faster than the Panther, and in miles per hour it happens that this speed difference is equal to twice the crew capacity of the Ridgback
- If you add up the total crew capacity of all three vehicles, the result is 13
- The Ridgback has a top speed of 56 mph, can carry three soldiers and hold one machine gun or a grenade launcher

# 4. A NATURAL DISASTER

You were taking part in a training exercise in Wales when your regiment, 21 Engineer Regiment, was informed of a major natural disaster that had occurred in the Caribbean, after which you were flown out to help provide aid. Two other regiments were also sent: 2 Medical Regiment and 17 Port and Maritime Regiment.

Can you work out in which order the different regiments arrived, and what they brought with them?

- One regiment brought blankets and tents, one brought water sanitation kits and another brought temporary fencing and tools
- The regiments bringing blankets and tents, and temporary fencing and tools arrived first and third respectively
- Your regiment did not arrive last
- 17 Port and Maritime Regiment brought water sanitation kits

# 5. INTERNATIONAL WORK

The British Army is active in many different places around the world, protecting Britain's allies and maintaining readiness to react to international events.

Soldiers Raj, Harry and Jinny have all been deployed abroad for the same length of time. Can you work out which countries they are deployed to, and how long their deployments are?

You will need to use some geographical knowledge to help you with this puzzle.

- Harry and Raj both left at the start of January
- Jinny is deployed in a British overseas territory 400 miles off the south-east coast of Argentina
- Jinny left in the middle of March, at which point Harry was halfway through his deployment
- Raj was deployed to the same place as the soldier who gets home in August
- Harry is deployed in a country bordering Mexico, whose first letter is 'B'

# PRACTICAL PUZZLES

## 1. LOSING THE LIGHT

You suspect that some images and navigation information that you have recently received from drone footage of a UK landing site are not accurate. This aerial photo has the timestamp 1800, 15/12/2018. From the positions of the shadows, how can you tell this is not a correct time stamp?

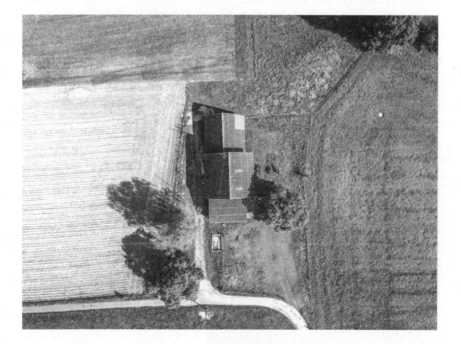

## 2. EMERGENCY NAVIGATION

A soldier has been deployed on exercise to southern Australia and has become detached from his section in the Outback. He does not have a map, compass or GPS at his disposal. He remembers from his exercise briefing that if he heads south, he will eventually get back to civilisation and rescue, but if he heads north, he will wander further into the Outback and almost certainly die of exposure.

Glancing at his watch he notes that it is 0900, 22 March. The image below shows the soldier from behind and the shadow he is casting on the ground. The soldier thinks back to the Emergency Navigation lesson he received in training at the Royal School of Military Survey.

He recalls the following facts:

- The sun is at its highest point in the sky at midday. At this time in the northern hemisphere, it will be to the south, and in the southern hemisphere it will be to the north
- The sun rises due east on only two days of the year, the equinoxes, near 22 March and 22 September each year
- The sun will travel across the sky at a rate of approximately 15 degrees per hour (since it travels 360 degrees around the Earth over a period of 24 hours)
- The sun rose at 0600 this morning

Based on these points, which direction is his shadow indicating and how should the soldier proceed relative to the shadow to travel south and make it to safety?

## 3. SENSIBLE SHADE

You need to urgently find a suitable place to conceal yourself in a compound to avoid enemy detection. It's just before sunrise, and you know from your training that, with no overhead cover available, it is better to hide in the shade of another building than in direct sunlight.

The time is 0630 and the date is 22 September. The sky is clear of clouds and you are in the UK. Which of the points marked 'x' on the map below would be the most appropriate for you to find cover in, when the sun rises?

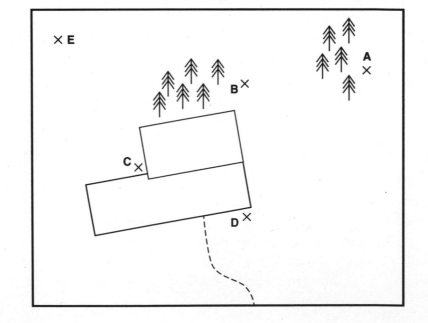

## 4. STICKS AND STONES

You have become separated from your unit and are now lost in a hot desert somewhere in the northern hemisphere, without a compass, map, GPS, smart device or any form of communication. There are no clouds and the sun is shining strongly.

You know that if you head due east you will eventually come to a settlement where you can make contact with your unit, so you need to work out which way is east.

The only items you have at your disposal are two small stones and a long, straight stick, all of which lie in the sand in front of you. You are confident that with these materials, and the following knowledge from your Emergency Navigation lessons, you can draw a line that will point you in the direction you need to walk.

All you need to solve this task is to remember that:

- The sun travels across the sky from east to west
- The sun casts shadows that fall in the opposite direction to the sun's location in the sky – so shadows will move from west to east as the day goes on

How can you accurately calculate the direction you must walk in?

## 5. SEARCH AREA

Your unit has been given orders to search multiple areas of open grassland, as you suspect there may be traps hidden by poachers in the terrain. The operation must be carried out quickly to avoid detection and consequent conflict. The best way to do this is to split up into groups, with each group searching areas of terrain of exactly the same size.

Below are the perimeters of the areas of grassland that must be searched. Can you draw along the grid lines to split each section into *four* identically shaped areas? Areas may be rotated, but cannot be reflections of one another (unless they also happen to be rotations too).

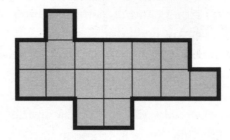

Once you have solved this puzzle, try these five further challenges, each of which gets progressively trickier.

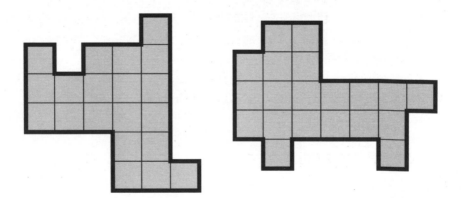

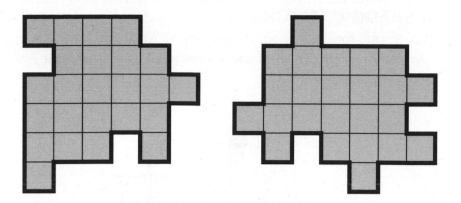

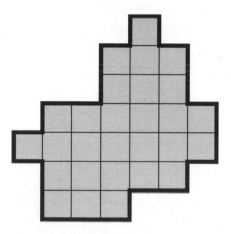

## 6. SHADOW MATCH

Can you work out which of the shadows below is being cast by the transmission mast?

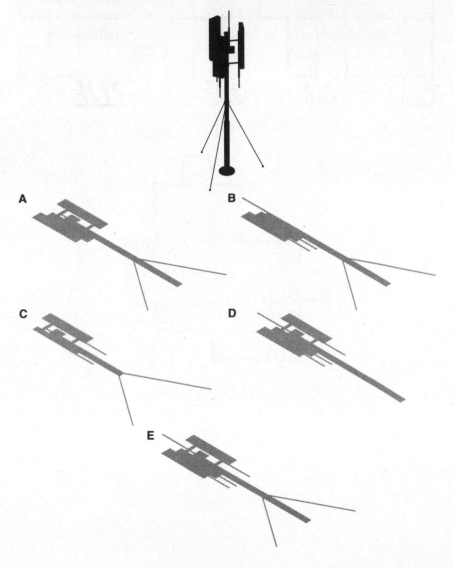

16

## 7. ON REFLECTION

You have taken cover underneath a rocky outcrop when you hear a vehicle approaching. From your position, you cannot see the vehicle, but a pool of water in front of you shows a reflection of the unknown truck, including the following reflected words on the surface of the water. What does it say?

MÉDECINS SANS FRONTIÈRES

# CAMOUFLAGE AND NIGHT VISION

## 1. RAPID DIFFERENCES

How quickly can you spot changes in your environment? In order to respond effectively to unidentified threats, you need to be alert and paying attention to small details, even those that may seem initially insignificant.

There are five differences between the image on this page and the one opposite. Can you find them all in under one minute?

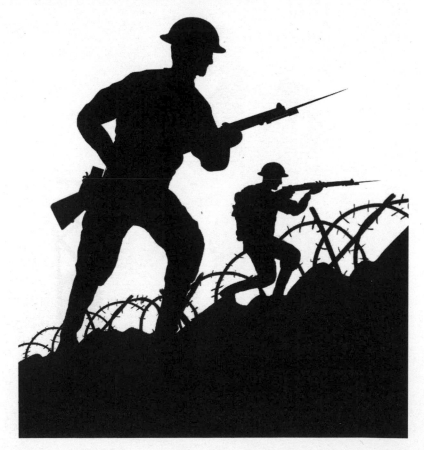

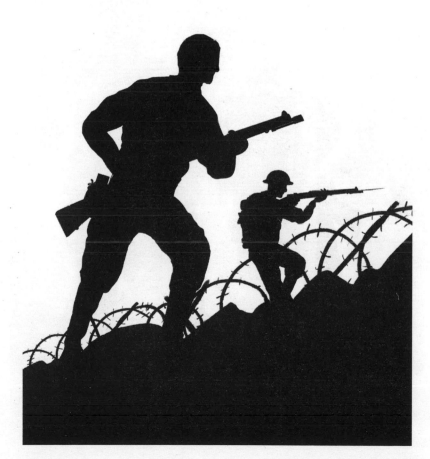

## 2. SUBTLER DIFFERENCES

Look closely. The following two images also have just five differences between them, but they may take you longer to spot than those on the previous page. Can you find them all in under five minutes?

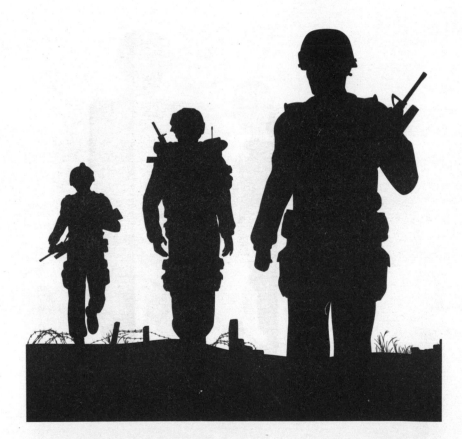

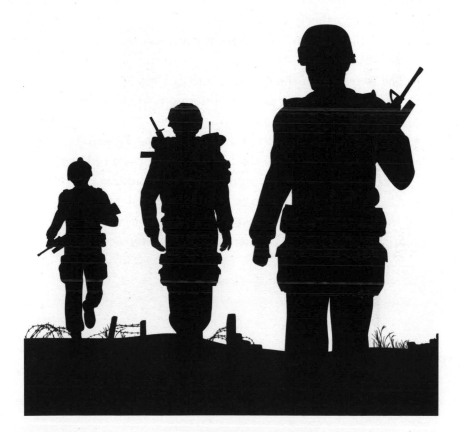

## 3. NIGHT NAVIGATION

Soldiers are taught to navigate at night in the northern hemisphere by locating Polaris, the Pole Star, also known as the North Star. Although it is extremely bright and therefore relatively easy to spot, its location can also be confirmed by using two other constellations: Cassiopeia; and the part of the constellation of Ursa Major, the Great Bear, known as the Plough.

Once you have located Polaris, you have found north – since it will be in a northerly direction from you. If you have trouble spotting it directly, you can locate it using one of these methods:

- The two stars at the opposite end of Ursa Major from its 'handle' are known as the pointer stars. They point to Polaris.
- If you hold your hands up in front of you, Polaris can be found roughly 2 hand spans from the bottom of Ursa Major in the direction pointed by the pointer stars.
- Also, a line from the tip of the 'handle' of Ursa Major to the end star on the flattest side of Cassiopeia (also the faintest star in that constellation) will intersect with Polaris.

These observations can be seen in this diagram:

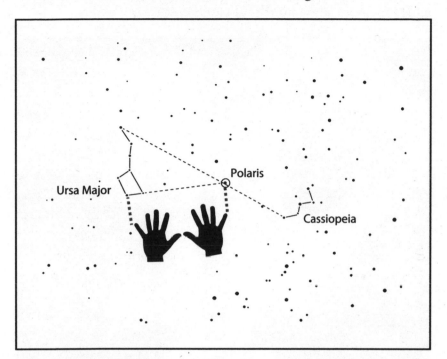

During night operations, however, a clear sky showing the whole constellation system cannot always be relied upon. Cloud cover must be taken into account. Using the above techniques, however, it is still possible to navigate north even when some of the stars are not visible.

Can you locate the position of Polaris in the picture below, which includes some unhelpful cloud cover?

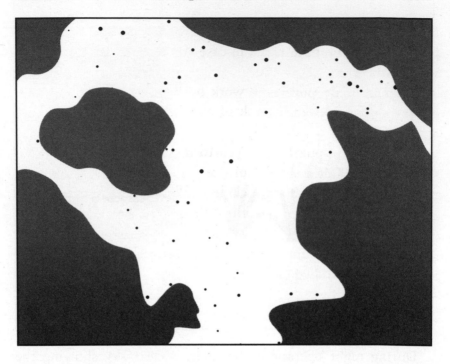

# MAZES AND NAVIGATION

It is important to be aware of your surroundings, and to remember the route you have taken in case you need to retreat via the same path.

Try these maze puzzles to work on your navigation skills. It can be difficult to keep track of a path while also navigating a maze.

The following puzzles ask you to count various things. You should only count a shape, turn or bridge if it is on the *direct* path to the exit. So, don't include any on side paths. This will require you to keep track both of the counts *and* whether you are retracing your path from a dead end.

Compare your counts for each maze against those given in the solutions. How did you do?

## 1. STAR MAZE

Find your way from the entrance at the top of the maze to the exit at the bottom. While finding your route out, keep a mental count of the number of times you pass directly through a star.

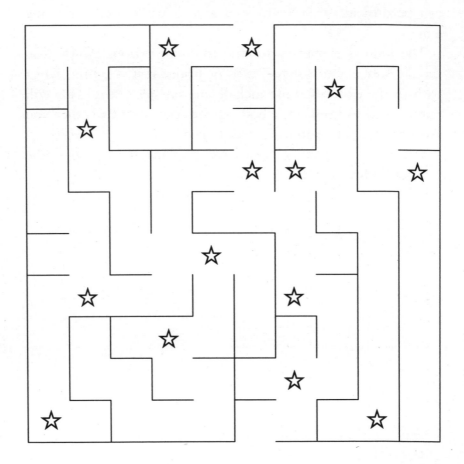

How many stars did you pass through?

## 2. LEFT-TURN MAZE

Find your way from the entrance at the top of the maze to the exit at the bottom. While finding your route out, keep a mental record of the number of times you make a left turn.

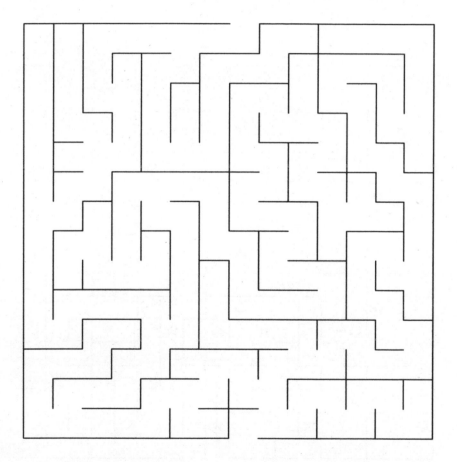

How many left turns did you make?

## 3. STARS AND DIAMONDS MAZE

Find your way from the entrance at the top of the maze to the exit at the bottom. While finding your route out, keep separate mental counts of the number of stars and number of diamonds you pass through.

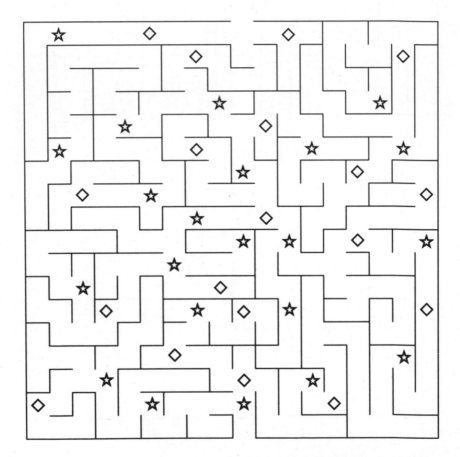

How many stars, and how many diamonds, did you pass?

# 4. LEFT- AND RIGHT-TURN MAZE

Find your way from the entrance at the top of the maze to the exit at the bottom. While finding your route out, keep separate mental counts of the number of left turns and right turns you make.

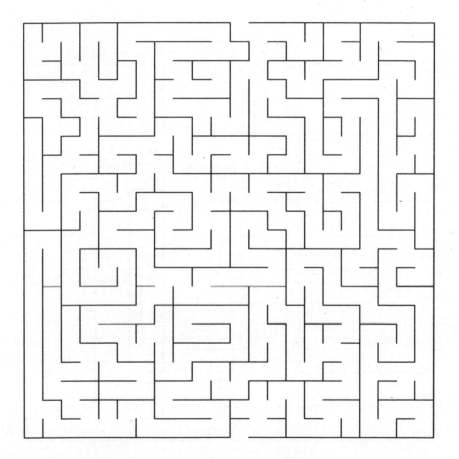

How many left turns did you make? How many right turns?

## 5. UNDER-BRIDGE MAZE

Find a path from the entrance at the top of the maze to the exit at the bottom. Your path may cross over or under itself, using the bridges in the maze. Can you keep track of how many bridges you cross *under* on your way through the maze?

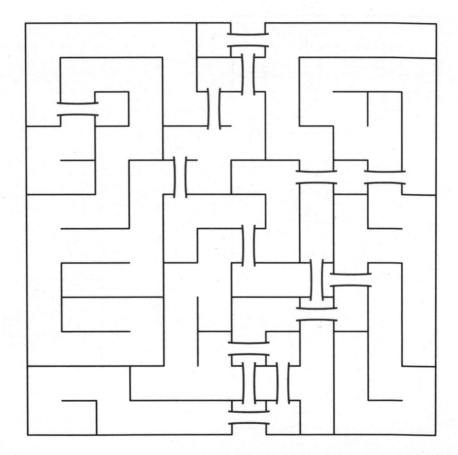

How many bridges did you cross under?

# 6. OVER-BRIDGE MAZE

Find a path from the entrance at the top of the maze to the exit at the bottom. Your path may cross over or under itself, using the bridges in the maze. Can you keep track of how many bridges you cross *over* on your way through the maze?

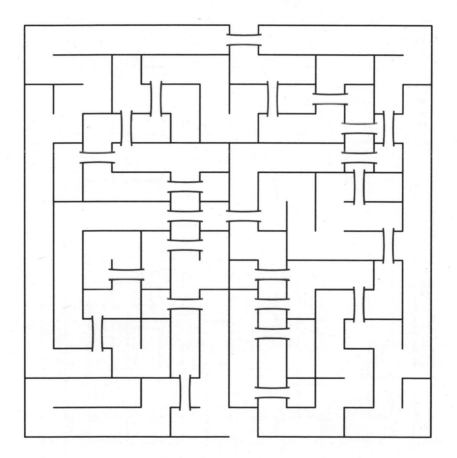

How many bridges did you cross over?

## 7. UNDER- AND OVER-BRIDGE MAZE

Find a path from the entrance at the top of the maze to the exit at the bottom. Your path may cross over or under itself, using the bridges seen in the maze. Can you keep track of the total number of bridges you cross either over or under, to exit the maze? Keep just one single total of both, but don't count a bridge more than once – so if you have already crossed over it, don't count it again if you go under it, and vice versa.

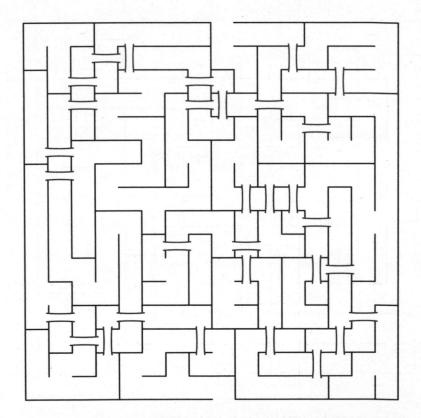

How many bridges did you cross *under* and *over* in total?

# 8. UNDER- OR OVER-BRIDGE MAZE

Find a path from the entrance at the top of the maze to the exit at the bottom. Your path my cross over or under itself, using the bridges seen in the maze. Can you keep track of how many bridges you cross *over*, and how many you cross *under*, to exit the maze?

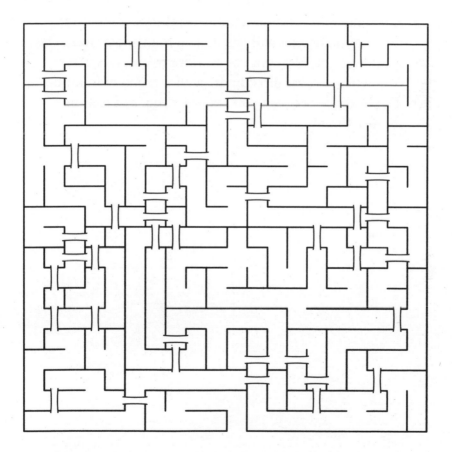

How many bridges did you cross *under*? How many *over*?

## 9. FIND YOUR SUPPLIES

You have been informed that supplies are being air-dropped into a location shown on the map opposite. Your current location is not marked, but you know you are due south of a point where a track and a road intersect. For security, the exact location of the drop has not been circulated, but you have been given the following clues:

- If you take the most direct route as the crow flies to the drop-off point, you will pass over a road and a river. This route will not, however, use a bridge to cross the river
- You will also pass directly through a group of buildings
- The distance between you and the drop, as the crow flies, is 10 km

1. Can you find your current location on the map, choosing from the locations labelled A–F?
2. Can you pinpoint the location of the supply drop, choosing from the locations labelled A–F?

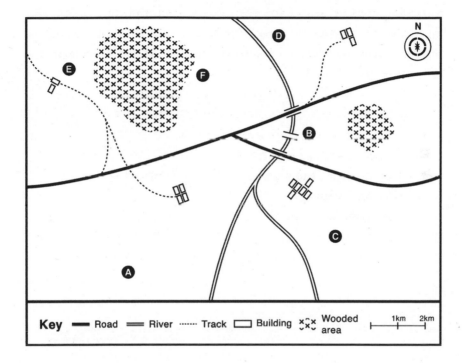

Key ▬ Road ═ River ⋯ Track ▭ Building ×ˣ× Wooded area    1km 2km

## 10. SETTING UP CAMP

You have been given the map opposite and asked to locate the best position for your unit to set up camp overnight. There are four suggested locations for a campsite, each marked 'X' on the map, and labelled from A to D. It is your job to decide which is the most suitable. You know from expedition training that the best campsites should ideally be:

- on level ground
- near or with access to a water supply
- accessible on foot and by road
- sheltered from the elements and not exposed (e.g., by being on a hilltop)
- away from large, permanent settlements

Using your map-reading skills, and the information opposite, can you determine which of the labelled locations is the most suitable to set up camp for the night?

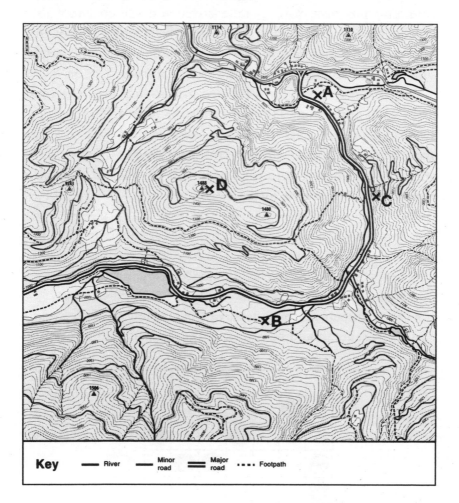

## 11. TENTS

Your unit has been told to take cover and set up camp in a wooded area overnight. You know that the weather will be dry, with clear skies and next to no wind, so camping is appropriate, with minimal risk of debris falling from the trees.

You have been given the following grid to help you determine where each of the makeshift tents must be placed. The circles in the grid represent trees that have been deemed safe to camp underneath. Each tree will have one tent erected next to it. In order to determine where each tent will be pitched, you have been given the following instructions:

- Tents must be pitched in squares that are horizontally or vertically adjacent to a tree square
- Tents must not be pitched in adjacent squares to other tents – not even diagonally
- The numbers on the outside of the grid tell you how many tents should be placed in that row or column

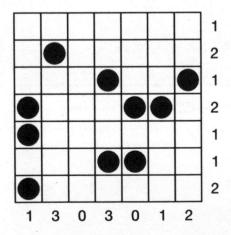

Once you've completed the first puzzle, try this tougher version:

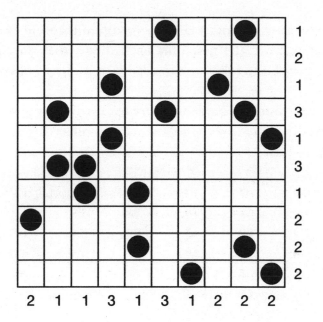

## 12. GRID REFERENCES – STANDARD

You have returned from a timed expedition training exercise to find that you are the first unit back. Later that day, you are presented with the following challenge as a means of congratulations.

Can you fill in the hidden picture to reveal your prize? Shade in squares indicated by the following grid references in order to claim it.

| | | | | | | | |
|---|---|---|---|---|---|---|---|
| B3 | G12 | I12 | H9 | E1 | A7 | F4 | E12 |
| J2 | A8 | G1 | F9 | B10 | E9 | L6 | A4 |
| K3 | D12 | D1 | L7 | C2 | L4 | H12 | J11 |
| L5 | L8 | G6 | L9 | A9 | A6 | C11 | G7 |
| G9 | G4 | G5 | G8 | F12 | I1 | A5 | K10 |
| H1 | F1 | E5 | | | | | |

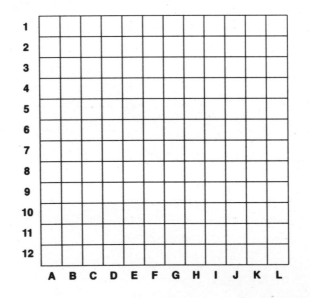

## 13. GRID REFERENCES – FOUR-DIGIT

In the army, soldiers are taught map-reading using a system of four-digit grid reference codes. Instead of a combination of letters and numbers as in the previous challenge, the numbers along the side and bottom of maps are combined to make one numerical grid reference.

The numbers along the horizontal axis are known as eastings, and the numbers on the vertical axis are known as northings.

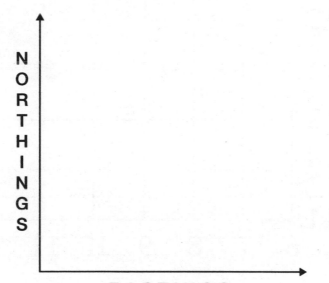

Where a grid reference is given, the first pair of digits is the easting, and the second pair is the northing. So, if you were given the grid reference 2256, you would find the 22 line on the easting axis, then find the point at which it crosses the 56 line on the northing axis. The grid reference will lead you to a point where two lines cross, and the square indicated by the reference is the one *north-east* of the crossing point.

For example, in the following grid, the shaded square would be indicated by the reference 1114:

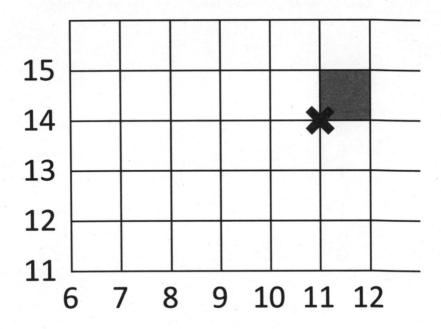

The easting is 11, the northing is 14, and the square to the north-east of the intersection is shaded.

With this in mind, can you shade in the squares indicated by the following grid references? You will reveal something you might find on an army uniform.

| | | | |
|---|---|---|---|
| 8735 | 8934 | 8535 | 8241 |
| 8142 | 9038 | 8136 | 9142 |
| 8937 | 9136 | 8238 | 8833 |
| 8732 | 8337 | 8836 | 8631 |
| 8340 | 8334 | 8634 | 8940 |
| 9041 | 8433 | 8637 | 8738 |
| 8235 | 8839 | 8532 | |
| 8436 | 9035 | 8538 | |
| 8439 | 9139 | 8139 | |

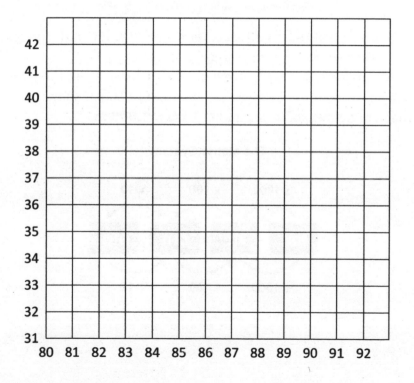

# MAP SCALES

In the military, soldiers are taught how to perform scale calculations in order to work out both the map and actual sizes of ground features.

In particular, soldiers are taught the GSM triangle:

**The GSM Triangle**

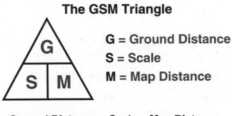

G = Ground Distance
S = Scale
M = Map Distance

**Ground Distance** = Scale x Map Distance
**Scale** = Ground Distance ÷ Map Distance
**Map Distance** = Ground Distance ÷ Scale

If any two of the distance components are known, the missing component of the triangle can be calculated.

All calculations in the army are carried out using the metric system. Conversion between different multipliers is shown in the diagram below; so, for example, 1 km = 1,000 m.

**The Metric System**

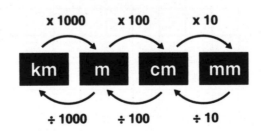

When carrying out any calculations with ground and map distance, it is critical that both components are first put into a common multiplier, i.e. distances must all be in the same units of measurement, before they can be used in calculation. In the following picture, for example, the distances in km and cm must both be converted into the same unit in order to calculate the scale. Here, they are both converted to metres, although, alternatively, one could have been converted to match the other:

### Calculate Scale

M = Map Distance = 40 cm
G = Ground Distance = 10 km
S = Map Scale?

- S = G ÷ M
- S = 10 km ÷ 40 cm
- S = 10,000 m ÷ 0.4 m
- S = 25,000

Map Scale = 1:25,000

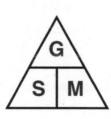

Using this information on how to calculate distance and scale, can you answer the following questions?

## 1. PHOTO INTELLIGENCE

Your unit has been tasked with conducting an attack on an enemy position. The Intelligence section provides you with an aerial photograph of the position, but doesn't tell you what scale it is. You notice there is a football pitch in the photo, which you know on average will measure 100 m in length. You measure the football pitch and it is 16 mm long in the photo. What is the approximate scale of the photo?

## 2. SCALE CALCULATIONS

Can you calculate these map scales based on the following map distances and ground distances? Remember to change at least one of the measurements to a common unit.

| | Map Distance | Ground Distance | Scale |
|---|---|---|---|
| a) | 20 cm | 60 km | _____ |
| b) | 50 mm | 250 m | _____ |
| c) | 4 cm | 8 km | _____ |
| d) | 14 mm | 5600 m | _____ |
| e) | 2.8 cm | 140 m | _____ |

# 3. GROUND-DISTANCE CALCULATIONS

Can you calculate these ground distances based on the following map distances and map scales? Give the ground distances in kilometres, or metres if less than 1 kilometre.

| | Map Distance | Scale | Ground Distance |
|---|---|---|---|
| a) | 3.7 cm | 1:25,000 | _____ |
| b) | 45 mm | 1:100,000 | _____ |
| c) | 8 cm | 1:40,000 | _____ |
| d) | 2.4 cm | 1:12,000 | _____ |
| e) | 38 mm | 1:250,000 | _____ |

# 4. MAP-DISTANCE CALCULATIONS

Can you calculate these map distances based on the following ground distances and map scales? Give the map distance in centimetres, or millimetres if less than 1 cm.

| | Ground Distance | Scale | Map Distance |
|---|---|---|---|
| a) | 2.8 km | 1:5,000 | _____ |
| b) | 450 m | 1:50,000 | _____ |
| c) | 7.5 km | 1:20,000 | _____ |
| d) | 700 m | 1:2,500 | _____ |
| e) | 32 km | 1:250,000 | _____ |

# CHAPTER 2

# COGNITIVE TESTING

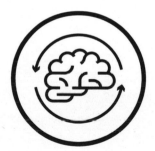

# COGNITIVE TESTS

Cognitive tests are valuable to a number of professions. Medical experts may use them to baseline and measure attention and memory in order to judge the cognitive health of a patient; Human Resource managers across industry may use them to assess the aptitude of prospective employees; those in education may use them to determine a child's current ability, before adapting the teaching they receive. Although the aim of these tests may be specific to the environment and those being tested, there is one common thread: a drive to ascertain how flexibly a person can think.

For the British Army, flexibility of mind is crucial. It enables our understanding of a situation, our environment, our adversaries and the opportunities we could take to be successful on military operations. Although we have world-class technology to support us, whether in our weapon systems, communications or the mechanisms by which we collect information on the enemy, we recognise that no army survives solely on the basis of its technological advantage. We have to be able to look at a problem or a mission in a variety of ways if we are to devise the most effective military plans, often in austere places where it would be inappropriate to deploy our most advanced systems.

Therefore, the greatest asset we have in our possession will always be our people. Furthermore, the variation with which people assess and approach tasks (because of differences in education, background and approaches to problems) gives us additional advantage, much needed for the diverse environments in which we operate.

The business of defence is fundamentally about understanding the threats to our peace and security and positioning ourselves to deal with them. This requires everything from a deep understanding of known enemies, to remaining vigilant for new threats, all the while adapting to meet the challenges presented. Change is our only constant and it takes huge intellectual agility not only to embrace it, but to use it to our advantage. Our ability to identify new dangers, learn quickly and apply our knowledge is essential to our decision making; in turn, making good decisions enables us to sustain the tempo of our operations. In sport, as in war, taking quick decisions, based on a sound assessment of changes in the situation, is what outsmarts the opposition and creates a battle-winning advantage.

The cognitive functions described above can be developed beyond the aptitude with which we are born. Training is crucial to military success, developing capabilities and putting our people in new situations in which they have to adapt. The tests in this chapter will ask you to perceive and consider a problem in different ways, to process and memorise information for later use, and to critically apply your knowledge, replicating the cycle of understanding, decision and action that army personnel experience. In pitting yourself against these puzzles, you will flex your cognitive abilities and realise that what we do and how we do it are very much dependent on keeping a lively, fully exercised mind.

Everyone's solved a puzzle at some point, whether it was in a magazine, computer game, phone app or something other. When you first try a new puzzle, you aren't sure how to go about solving it, but then, as you practise, you get better and better at it until, eventually, you know immediately how to get started on each new puzzle. But what if the puzzles were never familiar? In the army, you train for situations, but once you're actually in the field you'll always need to adjust to how things really are on the ground. So, in this chapter, we'll start with a regular puzzle that you may be familiar with, but then we'll continually change the rules. Can you adapt? Are you mentally flexible enough to cope with continual new challenges? It's time to find out.

# SUDOKU

In this section we'll start with a regular 9×9 sudoku puzzle and then we'll continually evolve it.

## 1. SUDOKU 9×9

You've probably tried, or at least seen, a sudoku puzzle before. The rules are simple:

- Place a single digit from 1 to 9 into each empty square
- No number can repeat in any row, column or bold-lined 3×3 box

Here's a standard sudoku. Can you solve it?

| 1 |   | 7 | 4 |   | 2 | 5 |   | 3 |
|---|---|---|---|---|---|---|---|---|
|   | 8 |   |   |   |   |   | 1 |   |
| 3 |   |   |   | 1 |   |   |   | 8 |
| 8 |   |   | 1 |   | 4 |   |   | 2 |
|   |   | 3 |   |   |   | 6 |   |   |
| 9 |   |   | 6 |   | 7 |   |   | 4 |
| 6 |   |   |   | 4 |   |   |   | 1 |
|   | 5 |   |   |   |   |   | 4 |   |
| 2 |   | 8 | 5 |   | 1 | 9 |   | 7 |

## 2. SUDOKU 6×6

Sudoku don't have to be 9x9. They can be any size square that isn't prime. (If it were prime, you wouldn't be able to draw any boxes in the grid.) Here's a 6×6 puzzle:

- Place a single digit from 1 to 6 into each empty square
- No number can repeat in any row, column or bold-lined 3×2 box

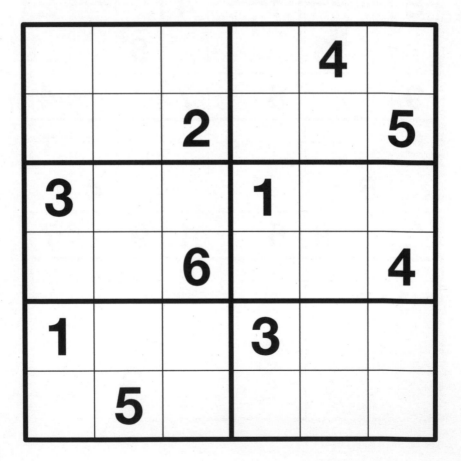

## 3. LATIN SQUARE

A sudoku puzzle has three different types of constraint: row, column and bold-lined box. If we remove the bold-lined boxes, we end up with what's known as a 'Latin square':

- Place a single digit from 1 to 6 into each empty square
- No number can repeat in any row or column

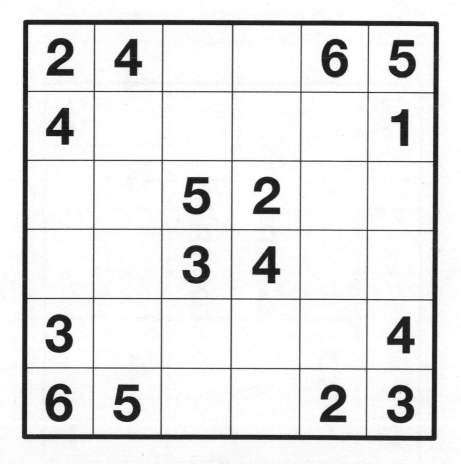

## 4. TOUCHY

Instead of boxes, we can add in other types of constraint. These help make the puzzle more interesting, and provide new challenges. In this puzzle, identical numbers can't touch diagonally (they already can't touch horizontally or vertically, since numbers can't repeat in a row or column):

- Place a single digit from 1 to 6 into each empty square
- No number can repeat in any row or column
- Identical numbers can't touch diagonally

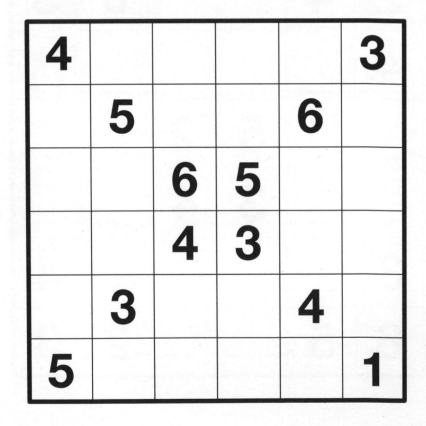

## 5. TOUCH SUDOKU

We can add the boxes back in too:

- Place a single digit from 1 to 6 into each empty square
- No number can repeat in any row, column or bold-lined 3×2 box
- Identical numbers can't touch, including diagonally

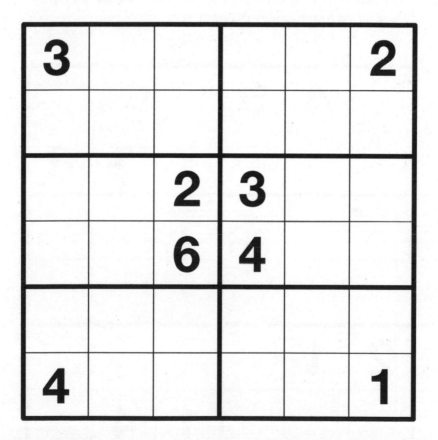

## 6. TWO-STEP DIAGONAL SUDOKU

We can also extend the no-touching rule, so squares that are two steps away diagonally also can't touch:

- Place a single digit from 1 to 6 into each empty square
- No number can repeat in any row, column or bold-lined 3×2 box
- Identical numbers can't appear in squares that are either one or two steps away diagonally

| | 4 | 6 | | | |
|---|---|---|---|---|---|
| | | | | 3 | 6 |
| | | | | | |
| | | | | | |
| 2 | 1 | | | | |
| | | | 1 | 4 | |

## 7. DIAGONAL SUDOKU

Instead of restricting numbers from touching one another diagonally in general, we can draw in diagonal extra regions where numbers can't repeat. In this puzzle, also known as 'sudoku-x', numbers can't repeat on the marked diagonal lines:

- Place a single digit from 1 to 6 into each empty square
- No number can repeat in any row, column, bold-lined 3×2 box or marked diagonal

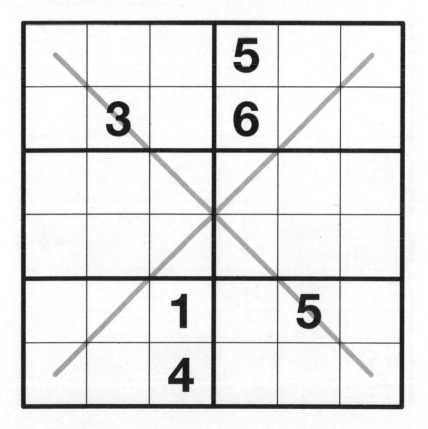

## 8. REGIONAL SUDOKU

We can replace the diagonal constraints with any other extra regions we like. In this puzzle, two extra shaded regions are present. Digits also can't repeat in these regions:

- Place a single digit from 1 to 6 into each empty square
- No number can repeat in any row, column, bold-lined 3×2 box or shaded region

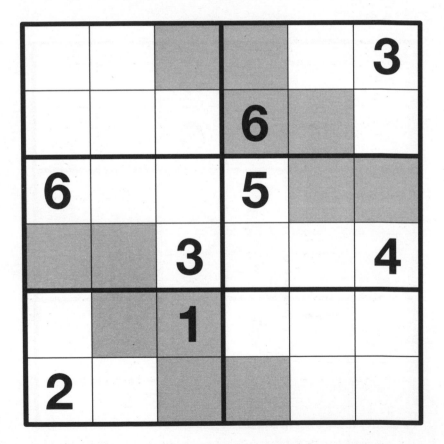

## 9. JIGSAW SUDOKU

Instead of adding extra, shaped regions, we can simply replace the boxes with *all* shaped regions. Most people find that this makes the puzzle feel much trickier, since it makes it tougher to scan the grid for deductions. Logically, however, it is no more complex:

- Place a single digit from 1 to 6 into each empty square
- No number can repeat in any row, column or bold-lined region

## 10. WRAP-AROUND SUDOKU

Once we have abandoned the fixed boxes, we can go a step further with our jigsaw-shaped regions, and allow them to 'wrap around' from one side of the grid to the other. In this puzzle, some regions continue across the ends of the puzzle. If there is no bold line to the side of the grid, then the same region continues on the opposite end of the same row or column.

- Place a single digit from 1 to 6 into each empty square
- No number can repeat in any row, column or bold-lined wrap-around region

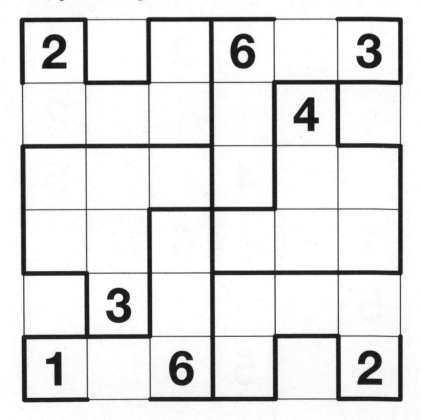

## 11. WRAP-AROUND BOXED SUDOKU

We can add one final touch by *also* adding in the boxes that we have in a regular sudoku. In this puzzle, every square has *four* different types of region covering it – a row, column, box and jigsaw region:

- Place a single digit from 1 to 6 into each empty square
- No number can repeat in any row, column, 3×2 box or bold-lined wrap-around region
- The six 3×2 boxes are indicated by continuous shaded/ unshaded areas

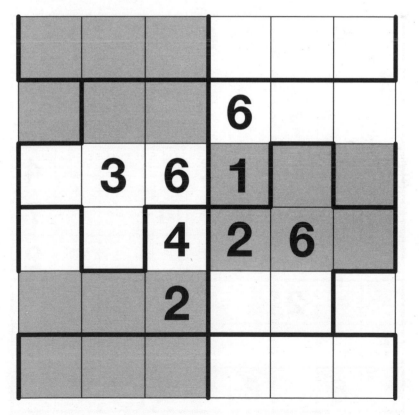

# REVENGE OF SUDOKU

Now that you've worked through the previous 11 puzzles, and seen how even small changes in a situation can create what feels like an entirely new scenario, let's start again from a regular sudoku – but this time use larger puzzles, and try an even more extensive set of variations.

## 1. SUDOKU

Here's a standard sudoku to start from:

|   | 8 |   | 4 | 6 | 7 |   | 9 |   |
|---|---|---|---|---|---|---|---|---|
| 1 |   |   |   |   |   |   |   | 3 |
|   | 7 |   |   |   |   | 4 |   |   |
| 8 |   |   |   | 2 |   |   |   | 4 |
| 2 |   |   | 1 | 5 | 4 |   |   | 7 |
| 4 |   |   |   | 7 |   |   |   | 2 |
|   |   | 2 |   |   |   | 8 |   |   |
| 5 |   |   |   |   |   |   |   | 6 |
|   | 6 |   | 8 | 1 | 2 |   | 7 |   |

## 2. OUTSIDE SUDOKU

The clues in a regular puzzle are written inside the grid, but what if we put them outside? In this puzzle, you have to insert the clues yourself:

- Place a single digit from 1 to 9 into each empty square
- No number can repeat in any row, column or bold-lined 3×3 box
- Digits outside the grid must be placed into one of the nearest three squares in their row or column – but not necessarily in the order given

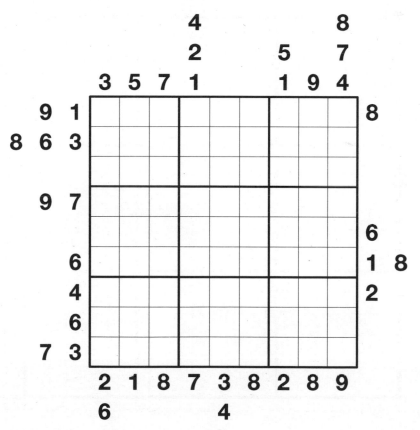

## 3. QUAD CLUE SUDOKU

There are other ways to start from a blank grid too. In this puzzle, the clues are written on the intersections of the grid lines, and it's up to you to add them to the puzzle:

- Place a single digit from 1 to 9 into each empty square
- No number can repeat in any row, column or bold-lined 3×3 box
- Digits on the intersection of four squares must be inserted, one each, into those four squares – but not necessarily in the order given

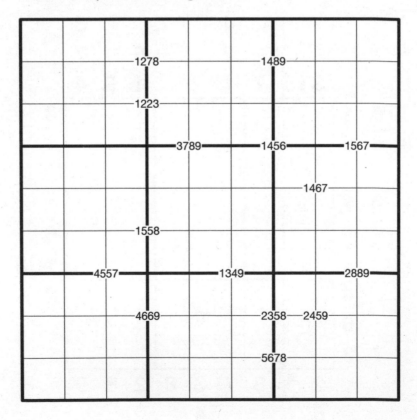

## 4. TRIO SUDOKU

We can also add constraints that limit what digits can fit into each square, as in this puzzle:

- Place a single digit from 1 to 9 into each empty square
- No number can repeat in any row, column or bold-lined 3×3 box
- Some squares contain extra symbols:
  - Squares with an inset square must contain 4, 5 or 6
  - Squares with an inset circle must contain 7, 8 or 9
  - All other squares must contain 1, 2 or 3

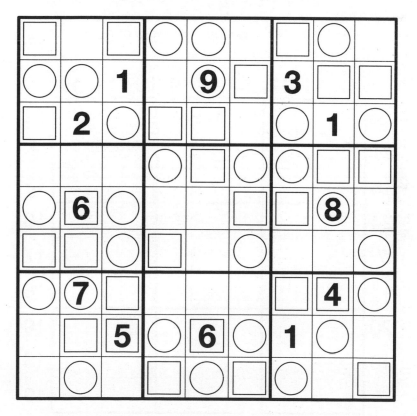

## 5. FRAME SUDOKU

Another way to vary the rules of sudoku is to use the actual values of the digits. In a normal sudoku puzzle, the digits could be any symbol – you could be placing symbols, shapes or letters and the puzzle wouldn't change. But what if we use the values of the digits as part of the puzzle?

Let's put the clues back outside the puzzle again, but this time we'll add a numerical constraint:

- Place a single digit from 1 to 9 into each empty square
- No number can repeat in any row, column or bold-lined 3x3 box
- Numbers outside the grid give the sum of the nearest three squares in their row or column

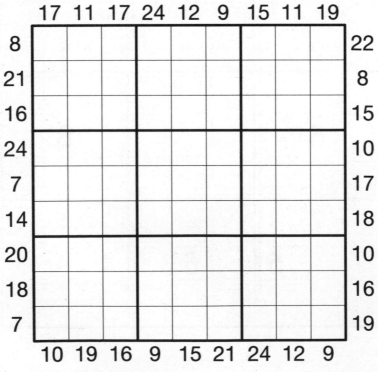

# 6. ARROW SUDOKU

We can also add sum-constraints within a puzzle too:

- Place a single digit from 1 to 9 into each empty square
- No number can repeat in any row, column or bold-lined 3×3 box
- Circled squares must contain a number equal to the sum of all the numbers along the length of their attached arrow

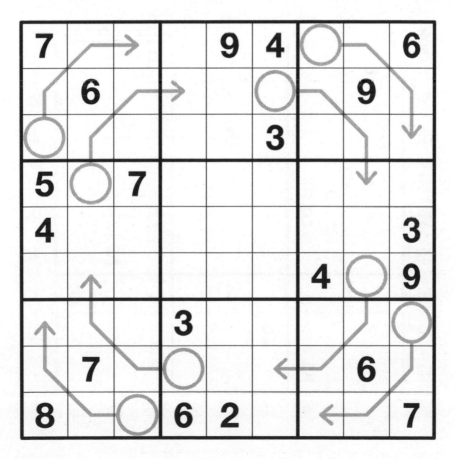

## 7. DIAGONAL-SUM SUDOKU

Sum arrows don't have to be inside the puzzle:

- Place a single digit from 1 to 9 into each empty square
- No number can repeat in any row, column or bold-lined 3×3 box
- Values outside the grid reveal the sum of all the numbers in the diagonal that they point to

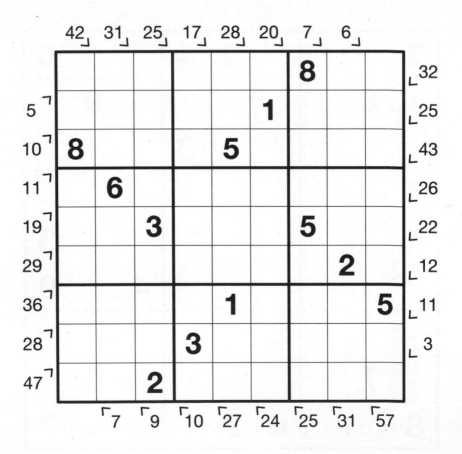

# 8. SUM SUDOKU

We can also add numerical constraints inside the grid, instead of outside:

- Place a single digit from 1 to 9 into each empty square
- No number can repeat in any row, column or bold-lined 3×3 box
- Values inside each inset cage must add up to the given total

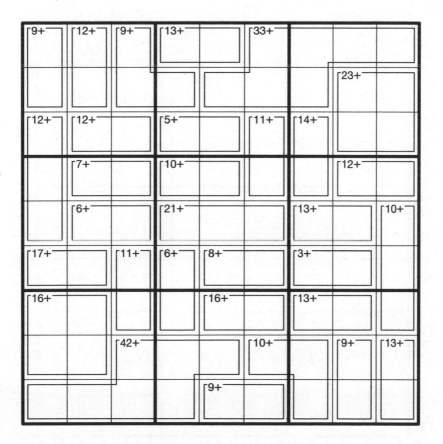

## 9. KILLER SUDOKU

We can also place additional constraints on the number cages we just added. This version of the puzzle is found in most newspapers, and is known as 'killer sudoku':

- Place a single digit from 1 to 9 into each empty square
- No number can repeat in any row, column or bold-lined 3×3 box
- Values inside each dashed-line cage must add up to the given total
- No number can repeat within any individual dashed-line cage

## 10. KILLER PRO SUDOKU

We don't need to stick just to addition. We can also allow subtraction, multiplication and division operations too:

- Place a single digit from 1 to 9 into each empty square
- No number can repeat in any row, column or bold-lined 3×3 box
- Values inside each dashed-line cage must result in the given value when the operation shown is applied between all the numbers in that cage. For subtraction and division operations, start with the largest value in the cage and then subtract/divide by the remaining values in any order
- No number can repeat within any individual dashed-line cage

## 11. MYSTERY KILLER PRO SUDOKU

Now it's up to you, when solving, to work out whether the rule for each cage is to add, subtract, multiply or divide:

- Place a single digit from 1 to 9 into each empty square
- No number can repeat in any row, column or bold-lined 3×3 box
- Values inside each dashed-line cage must result in the given value when you either add, subtract, multiply or divide all the numbers in the cage. For subtraction and division operations, start with the largest value in the cage and then subtract/divide by the remaining values in any order
- No number can repeat within any individual dashed-line cage

# 12. KILLER SUDOKU 0-8

Returning to the basic 'killer sudoku' puzzle type, now that the digits are being used for their values, we can also mix up the puzzle by changing the values of the digits that we use:

- Place a single digit from 0 to 8 into each empty square
- No number can repeat in any row, column or bold-lined 3×3 box
- Values inside each dashed-line cage must add up to the given total
- No number can repeat within any individual dashed-line cage

## 13. MYSTERY KILLER PRO SUDOKU 0–8

If we then allow addition, subtraction, multiplication and division, *and* hide the clues for these, we end up with a much tougher version of sudoku:

- Place a single digit from 0 to 8 into each empty square
- No number can repeat in any row, column or bold-lined 3×3 box
- Values inside each dashed-line cage must result in the given value when you either add, subtract, multiply or divide all the numbers in the cage. For subtraction and division operations, start with the largest value in the cage and then subtract/divide by the remaining values in any order
- No number can repeat within any individual dashed-line cage

# UNEQUAL SUDOKU

In the previous section, we explored what happens if you allow the digits in a sudoku puzzle to use their values more meaningfully than as just abstract symbols. In this section, we'll try changing the puzzle in completely different ways that *also* take advantage of this.

## 1. FUTOSHIKI

We won't start with sudoku at all this time. In this sort of puzzle, commonly found in newspapers, the aim is to obey the inequality arrows:

- Place a single digit from 1 to 6 into each empty square
- No number can repeat in any row or column
- Inequality symbols between some pairs of squares point to the square with the lower value of the two

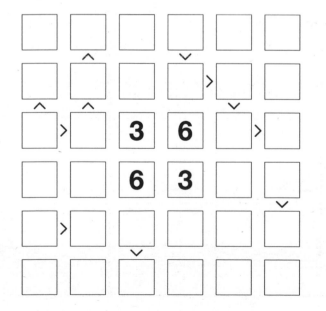

## 2. FULL FUTOSHIKI

Since numbers can't repeat in a row or column, there's no reason why we cannot mark in inequality signs between *every* pair of neighbouring squares. It makes the puzzle logically simpler, but it also acts like camouflage and makes it harder to spot the next deduction:

- Place a single digit from 1 to 6 into each empty square
- No number can repeat in any row or column
- Inequality symbols between pairs of squares point to the square with the lower value of the two

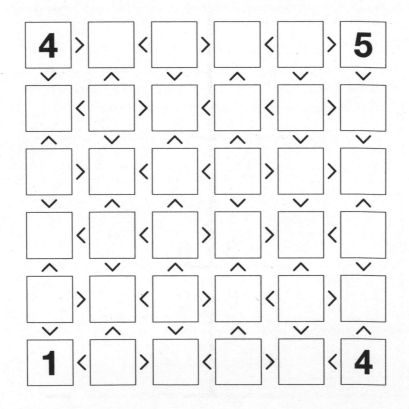

# 3. FULL INEQUALITY SUDOKU

Futoshiki is essentially a Latin square with added inequality constraints. We can instead add those inequality constraints to regular sudoku:

- Place a single digit from 1 to 6 into each empty square
- No number can repeat in any row, column or bold-lined 3×2 box
- Inequality symbols between pairs of squares point to the square with the lower value of the two

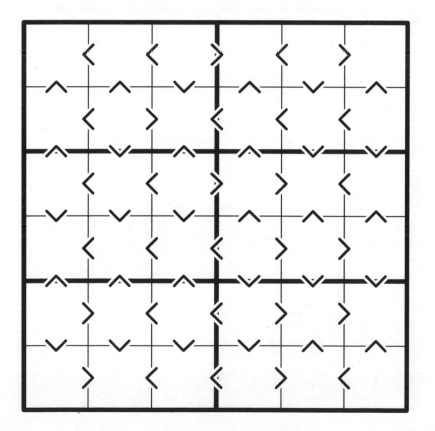

## 4. INEQUALITY SUDOKU

As with Futoshiki, the puzzle is arguably a little easier to make sense of when there are fewer inequalities:

- Place a single digit from 1 to 6 into each empty square
- No number can repeat in any row, column or bold-lined 3×2 box
- Inequality symbols between some pairs of squares point to the square with the lower value of the two

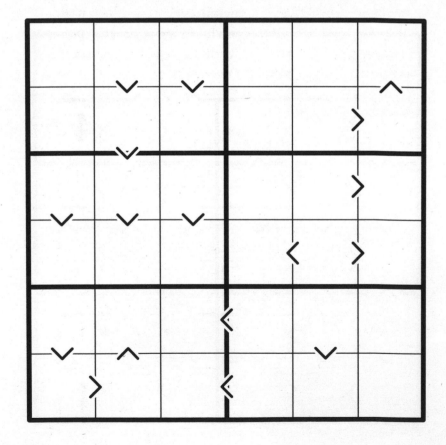

## 5. QUAD-MAX SUDOKU 6×6

Filling the puzzle with inequality signs doesn't make for a particularly fun solve, particularly as the grid gets larger. One way to avoid this is to look for more interesting inequality relationships:

- Place a single digit from 1 to 6 into each empty square
- No number can repeat in any row, column or bold-lined 3×2 box
- If a square contains a value that is greater than the three squares touching its corner, including the diagonally touching square, then it includes an arrow that points at that corner (so a square with all four arrows contains a value that is higher than *every* square it touches)

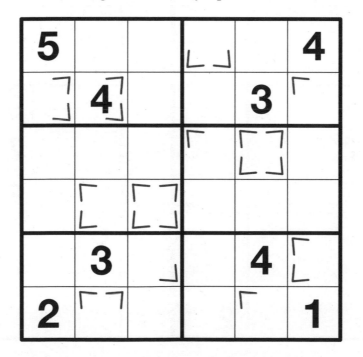

## 6. QUAD-MAX SUDOKU 9×9

We can also use inequalities in a regular-size puzzle:

- Place a single digit from 1 to 9 into each empty square
- No number can repeat in any row, column or bold-lined 3×3 box
- If a square contains a value that is greater than the three squares touching its corner, including the diagonally touching square, then it includes an arrow that points at that corner (so a square with all four arrows contains a value that is higher than *every* square it touches)

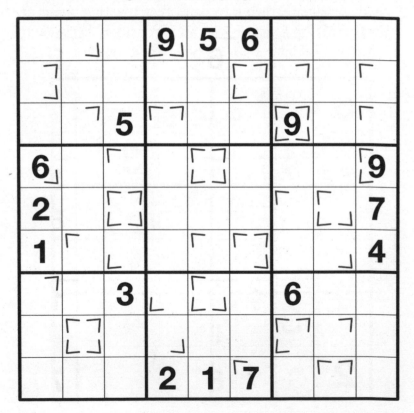

# 7. THERMOMETER SUDOKU

A much more elegant way to present an inequality puzzle is with thermometers:

- Place a single digit from 1 to 9 into each empty square
- No number can repeat in any row, column or bold-lined 3×3 box
- Values on a thermometer must increase at each step of the thermometer, increasing from the bulb up to the tip of the thermometer ('increase' means they must be greater, so a thermometer could, for example, contain 2379, but not 2279)

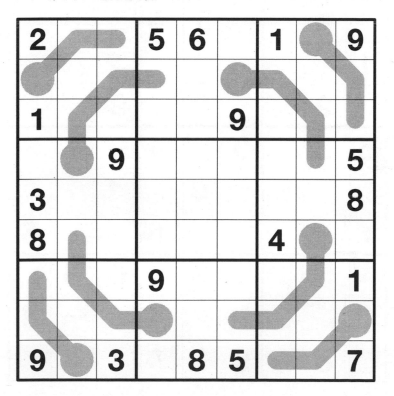

## 8. CREASING SUDOKU

We can create a new variant of sudoku by hiding the thermometer bulbs:

- Place a single digit from 1 to 9 into each empty square
- No number can repeat in any row, column or bold-lined 3×3 box
- Values on a thermometer must increase at each step of the thermometer, increasing from one end to the other. It's up to you to work out which is the low end, and which is the high end

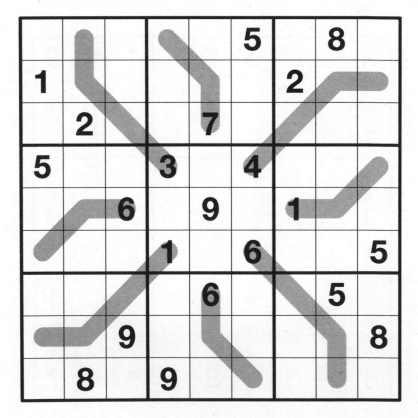

## 9. WORM SUDOKU

We can further restrain the inequalities by also specifying that values must be consecutive. Consecutive numbers are those with a numerical difference of 1, such as 2 and 3, or 7 and 8:

- Place a single digit from 1 to 9 into each empty square
- No number can repeat in any row, column or bold-lined 3×3 box
- Values on a worm must decrease by one at each step along the body of the worm, from its head (marked with eyes) all the way to its tail. (So, a four-square-long worm could have the values 8765 along it, but not 8764.)

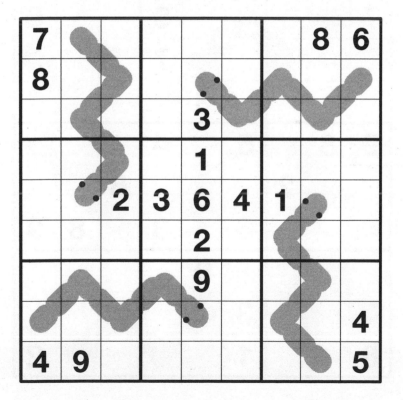

## 10. HEADLESS WORM SUDOKU

Just as with the creasing sudoku on page 86, we can stop marking the heads of the worms, to make it trickier:

- Place a single digit from 1 to 9 into each empty square
- No number can repeat in any row, column or bold-lined 3×3 box
- Values on a worm must decrease by one at each step along the body of the worm, from its head all the way to its tail – but it's up to you to work out which end is the head, and which end is the tail

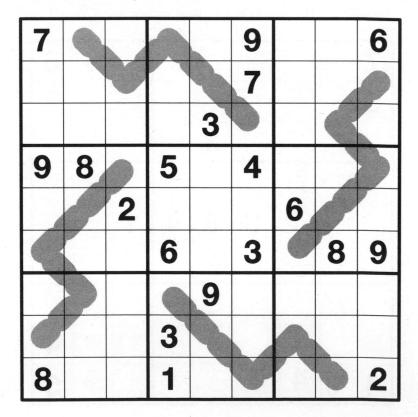

## 11. SNAKE SUDOKU

If we remove the inequality constraints, we can end up with a new type of puzzle:

- Place a single digit from 1 to 9 into each empty square
- No number can repeat in any row, column or bold-lined 3×3 box
- Values in neighbouring squares along the body of each snake must always be consecutive (so, for example, the values 345456 along the body of a snake would be valid, but 346789 would not be)

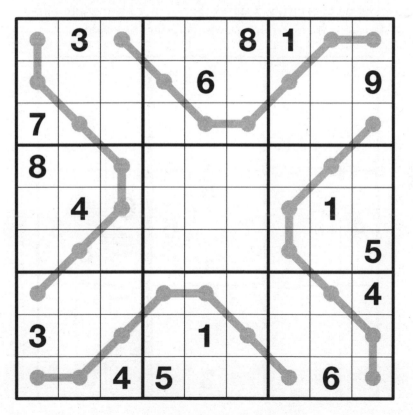

## 12. CONSECUTIVE SUDOKU

Snake sudoku is visually quite interesting, but we can keep the same concept and simply mark *all* neighbouring pairs of squares that contain consecutive values:

- Place a single digit from 1 to 9 into each empty square
- No number can repeat in any row, column or bold-lined 3×3 box
- *All* values in neighbouring squares (i.e. touching left/right/up/down) that are consecutive are marked with white bars
- Any neighbouring squares that do not have white bars between them *do not* contain consecutive values

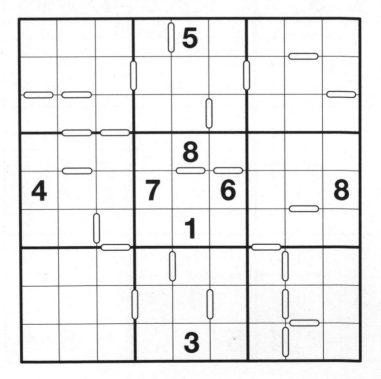

## 13. KROPKI SUDOKU

We can add on further value-based constraints. In this puzzle, we add to consecutive sudoku:

- Place a single digit from 1 to 9 into each empty square
- No number can repeat in any row, column or bold-lined 3×3 box
- Neighbouring squares with a white dot between them must contain consecutive values
- Neighbouring squares with a black dot between them must contain numbers where one is exactly twice the value of the other
- Neighbouring squares *without* either a white or black dot between them *do not* contain consecutive values or have one value equal to exactly twice the other

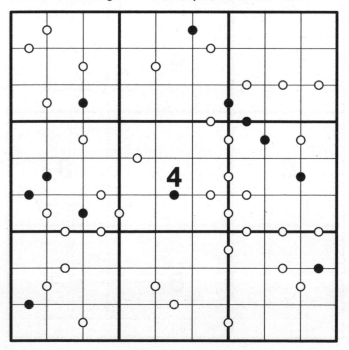

## 14. XV SUDOKU

Once we start marking relationships between neighbouring squares, there are all kinds of constraints we can add. For example, Roman numerals:

- Place a single digit from 1 to 9 into each empty square
- No number can repeat in any row, column or bold-lined 3×3 box
- Neighbouring squares with a 'V' between them must sum to 5 (such as 1 and 4)
- Neighbouring squares with a 'X' between them must sum to 10 (such as 3 and 7)
- Neighbouring squares *without* either a 'V' or 'X' between them must sum to any value other than 5 or 10

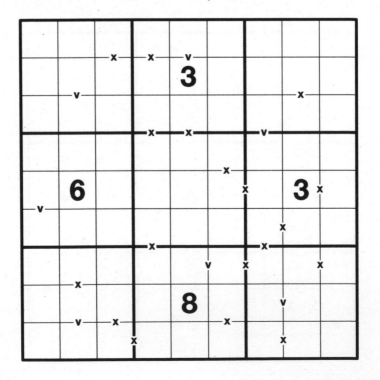

## 15. ANTI-XV SUDOKU

We can also use the absence of relationship markers to vary puzzles too:

- Place a single digit from 1 to 9 into each empty square
- No number can repeat in any row, column or bold-lined 3×3 box
- Neighbouring squares *never* contain values that sum to either 5 or 10

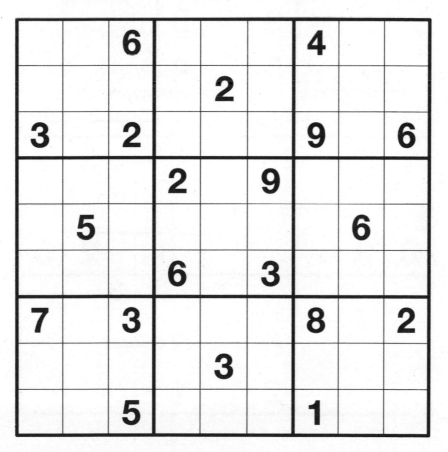

## 16. NON-CONSECUTIVE SUDOKU

We can do the same thing with consecutive markers too:

- Place a single digit from 1 to 9 into each empty square
- No number can repeat in any row, column or bold-lined 3×3 box
- Neighbouring squares *never* contain consecutive values, such as 3 and 4

| | | | 3 | | 8 | | | |
|---|---|---|---|---|---|---|---|---|
| | | | 5 | | 4 | | | |
| | | | | | | | | |
| 1 | 5 | | | | | | 3 | 7 |
| | | | | | | | | |
| 6 | 3 | | | | | | 2 | 5 |
| | | | | | | | | |
| | | | 6 | | 3 | | | |
| | | | 2 | | 1 | | | |

## 17. SUDOKU

And then, with one last rule change, we can return to regular sudoku again:

- Place a single digit from 1 to 9 into each empty square
- No number can repeat in any row, column or bold-lined 3×3 box

| | 7 | | | | | | 3 | |
|---|---|---|---|---|---|---|---|---|
| 8 | | | 6 | | 3 | | | 5 |
| | | 5 | 7 | | 9 | 8 | | |
| | 3 | 8 | | | | 2 | 4 | |
| | | | | 2 | | | | |
| | 4 | 7 | | | | 9 | 5 | |
| | | 6 | 9 | | 4 | 5 | | |
| 4 | | | 5 | | 2 | | | 8 |
| | 9 | | | | | | 6 | |

# AND FINALLY

Without checking back, can you say what property the number of puzzles in each section of this chapter shared?

# CHAPTER 3

# [ TEAMWORK ]

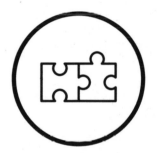

# TEAMWORK

# TEAM BUILDING

The power of the team sits at the very heart of what makes the British Army an effective and successful organisation. Teamwork presents a chance to deliver a result that is far greater than the sum of its parts, since each member has the ability to contribute their strengths to harness an effect that can be unstoppable! For this reason, the ability to build teams is considered very important and is one of the three pillars of army leadership. It is balanced and considered carefully alongside the need to achieve the task and the need to also develop individuals.

Creating and maintaining a good team is often considered by many leaders and organisations to be a difficult thing to achieve. However, the army believes differently; it can be achieved with some hard work and the consideration of a few simple rules. They are as follows:

1. Understand what you are trying to achieve. What is it as a team you are trying to work towards? This is often, though not necessarily, decided by the leader of the group. It needs to be clearly explained to all members of the team in a simple manner so that everyone understands and can contribute their ideas to the plan.

If other members can't explain it to each other in one or two sentences then it's probably too complicated or confusing.

2. Build a team identity. Consider what is common and good about your team: what makes you the same and is something you can all relate to? Now take those elements and nurture and invest time in them to develop the bonds between you and encourage commitment. You will see a change in those around you as they start to think more about the team identity and realise that they are part of something greater than themselves. The British Army uses its regimental groupings and other activities such as sports to build a strong identity.

3. Include others and seek out diversity in all its forms. Individuals will only commit to the team and its goals if they feel welcome and involved. Everyone will bring an idea, a strength or a skill to the team to help solve collective problems or make good decisions. These combined strengths can overcome what would be critical weaknesses. However, such diversity can only contribute where opinion can flourish and is listened to and respected by all. Such an environment will breed trust in the team and that trust will breed success.

4. Always seek to improve. When you have done well as a team, be prepared to think about how you can do better. Capture and remember what it was that worked, but be humble and inquisitive enough to consider what elements of the team's performance could be improved and what the route to excellence looks like for the team. Now break that excellence down into achievable targets and start hitting those targets.

5. Think about cooperation before control. In certain difficult situations, a team may need to be controlled by one of its members or the chosen leader to be effective. However, the most successful teams are those that look to cooperate first. They encourage initiative, creativity, and the confidence to act when an opportunity presents itself. If the team thinks first about control, then these positive conditions will be stifled. If you are the leader of the team, being cooperative rather than controlling will feel uncomfortable. Take a chance, embrace cooperation and prepare to be surprised by what your team will achieve.

Good luck!

# COMMAND AND LEADERLESS TASKS

The following challenges are designed to test your ability to work in a team. You will need to be a good communicator, be physically agile and use your logic and reasoning skills. You'll also need to keep calm under pressure, since your team members are relying on you. Some of the challenges will also involve a test of memory, so make sure you are paying attention from start to finish.

The challenges are split into two sections:

- Command tasks
- Leaderless tasks

Most of the command tasks require a leader or instruction-giver, who you can select from your team. It will be their job to guide the team through the challenge. The leaderless tasks – as the name suggests – have no leader and must be completed by all team members, each taking on a fair share of the work.

All the challenges have:

- An **objective** – which tells you the overall aim of the challenge
- A suggested **time limit** – but you can adjust this based on your team's skill level
- A suggested **team size**, although you can still try the tasks even if you don't have a team of the given size
- An **equipment** list. If you can't find all the items on the list, see if you can find reasonable substitutes. Some challenges already have substitutes suggested
- **Instructions** – which tell you what to do

- **Discussion** points – for you and your team to reflect on how the challenge went. There are no right answers to the questions they ask, but they are designed to make you think about your team-building skills
- An **expert challenge** – designed to make the challenge more difficult, and including tougher versions if you want to try the task again in the future

Some challenges also have hints at the end, below the expert challenges, in case your team is having difficulty.

You might not complete every challenge the first time you try it, but the experience of having a go will still be worthwhile – and you can then think about what you might do differently the next time. As an initial tip, remember that good teamwork involves listening as well as doing! No matter how good you are individually, if you can't communicate as a team then you won't be working as efficiently as you could be.

# COMMAND TASKS

## 1. SPAGHETTI BRIDGE

**Objective:** To build a bridge strong enough to bear a 1 kg weight.

*You will need*:

- 500 g of spaghetti
- A roll of sticky tape
- A 1 kg bag of flour (or something of equivalent shape and weight)
- Two chairs

*Suggested time limit*: 45 minutes
*Suggested team size*: 3 to 6 people

**Instructions**
You and your team must build a bridge that can hold the weight of a 1 kg bag of flour. The only materials you have at your disposal are 500 g of spaghetti and a roll of sticky tape. To test the bridge, you'll need two chairs placed 50 cm apart. The bridge should span the gap across the middle with enough extra space on both sides for it to rest safely.

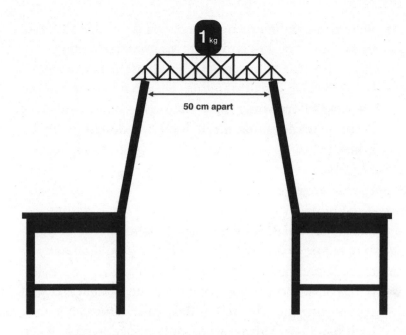

Your bridge can be of any shape or design, but can only be constructed with the two building materials provided. The bridge must be able to hold the bag of flour for 10 seconds, without any part of the bridge breaking, for the challenge to be completed. It also must stay sufficiently level that the flour does not fall off.

When your bridge is ready for testing, place the bag of flour in the *middle* of the bridge. You can place it down as gently as you like, but you must let go of it in order to test your bridge properly.

### Discussion points

- What worked well about your design? Is there anything you could have done differently, now that you've built your first spaghetti bridge?
- Did anyone take the lead when discussing how to build the bridge? If so, was this helpful?

- Were there any moments where you were able to learn from your mistakes and adapt your construction methods while you were still building the bridge?
- If your bridge is still standing, what happens if you place the bag of flour somewhere else on it – does it still hold? If not, what does that mean about the design of your bridge?

## Expert challenges

- If the bridge is still standing, you could try adding additional weights. How much weight can the bridge take before it starts to collapse? Can it hold an entire extra bag of flour?
- If you have successfully completed the challenge once, try splitting into two teams next time. The teams must each build two halves of the same bridge, which, when combined, can hold the weight of one bag of flour. You must split the 500 g of spaghetti between you, but you can have two rolls of sticky tape if you wish. You should avoid looking at the other team's half of the bridge during construction, but you can speak to each other. (You might want to create a barrier between the teams so that they can't see what the other team is building.) When both teams have completed their halves of the bridge, you have five minutes to join the two halves together to make one complete bridge. Test the strength of the bridge in the same way you tested the first one. How does it compare?

*Hint: a good bridge is designed so that the load-bearing is evenly distributed around all areas of the bridge. That means that although you'll be placing your bag of flour in the middle of the bridge, all parts should contribute to supporting the weight.*

## 2. BLIND DRAWING

**Objective:** To describe a picture seen only by you sufficiently well that a teammate can draw an exact copy.

*You will need*:

- Some paper
- A pen

*Suggested time limit*: 5 minutes
*Suggested team size*: 2+

### Instructions

This challenge can be completed with a minimum of two people. One person in the team chooses a picture from the page overleaf to describe to their teammate(s), and the other members of the team must then draw a copy of the picture as accurately as possible, based only on a verbal description given by their teammate. Start by deciding which person is going to describe the image; everyone else should then draw. Make sure no one sees anyone else's picture.

This challenge is designed to test your communication skills, so think carefully about what you want to say. The people drawing the images may *not* use an eraser, so descriptions should be as accurate as possible on the first attempt. The people drawing are allowed to ask the describer questions, if they are unclear on what has been said.

The images are taken from a standard set of symbols devised for joint military use by NATO. They will often appear in colour variations to denote the affiliation (friendly, hostile, neutral or unknown), but appear without colour here.

When the describer has finished describing the image, or when the time limit is up, everyone shows their drawings, and the describer shows the original image. How close did each drawer get?

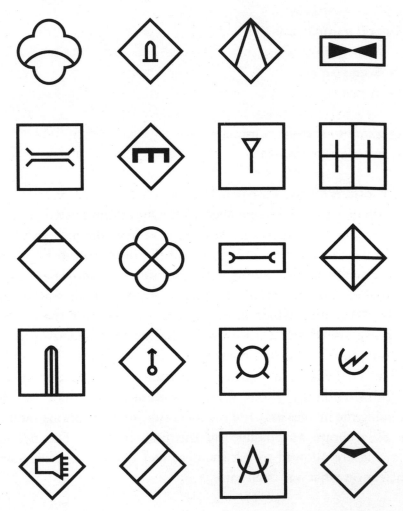

## Discussion points

- Do you think it's harder to draw or describe? Why? Are some people better at one task than the other?
- Is there anything you could have done differently? If so, try again with a different image.
- What did you learn about your own communication skills?

## Expert challenges

- Pick a simple image from a magazine or newspaper to describe, instead of one of those given on the previous page.
- Try describing the picture without using the words 'circle', 'square', 'triangle', 'rectangle' or 'line'.
- Can you still complete the challenge effectively if the people drawing are not allowed to speak, or ask any questions?
- Can you draw competitively against another team? Split into pairs, with one person in each pair able to see the image they are going to describe. They should both be describing the same image. Repeat the challenge in the same way as the first attempt. When all the teams have finished, or the time limit is up, compare your results. Which team's drawing is the most accurate? Did you notice anything about the methods the describers used to communicate the image? Were their methods different, and did that affect the result?

## 3. MINEFIELD

**Objective:** To cross the minefield, avoiding any casualties.

*You will need*:

- Some beanbags or cushions
- A blindfold
- Access to a large area, perhaps outside

*Suggested time limit*: Two minutes per teammate crossing the minefield

*Suggested team size*: 2–6

### Instructions

Place a number of soft objects, like cushions or beanbags, on the floor. They should be placed at least 2 metres from one another with enough space to walk around in between them. Each cushion or beanbag is now a mine, and the whole area is a minefield. Make sure there is nothing in the minefield that might cause harm if a teammate were to trip over, other than the cushions/beanbags themselves.

Mark out two clear areas, one on each side of the minefield, that are safe ground. Your task is now to guide each blindfolded team member from one side of the field to the other without them detonating any mines. They cannot touch any mine with any part of their body.

For each person crossing the minefield, one person should be nominated to be the team's guide. They will then give instructions on how to safely cross the minefield. If you are the guide, you can tell your teammate how many steps to walk forward in a straight line, and then which way to turn using 90-degree turns. An example might be: 'Take four steps forward, then turn 90 degrees to the left.'

When a person has safely reached the other side without touching any mines, someone else puts on the blindfold and repeats the task for another person who is yet to cross the minefield. If playing with more than two people, you can either have the same guide for every teammate crossing the field (until it is the guide's turn, themselves, to cross) or nominate a fresh guide for each new person crossing.

You should allow two minutes for each teammate to be guided across the field. If you are nominating a new guide between crossings, you must do this within the two-minute time limit. You can pass the blindfold from side to side of the minefield without worrying about detonating mines.

### Discussion points
- What did it feel like to be blindfolded and completely reliant on your teammates to keep you safe?
- Did you prefer to be guided through the minefield, or to be the one giving instructions? Why?
- Did the time pressure affect your ability to give instructions? If yes – how?

### Expert challenge
- Place the mines closer together or add more mines to the minefield.
- In larger groups, everyone should have one go at giving instructions to a blindfolded team member. Can you guide them across safely without discussing your instruction plan beforehand?

- Try having everyone in a larger group take it in turns to give directions to the blindfolded person, one instruction at a time.
- The original exercise allows time for the blindfolded team member to stop after turning. Can you still guide them through the minefield if they cannot stop and must always be walking at the same pace?

## 4. ELECTRIC GAP

**Objective:** To pass at least one team member through a gap in an electric fence without any casualties.

*You will need*

- A plastic hula hoop
- Two ropes, each 2 metres in length (skipping ropes will suffice)

*Suggested time limit*: 15 minutes
*Suggested team size*: 6

**Instructions**
Your team has come across a gap in an electric fence, which at least one member of the team must pass through to complete the challenge. To create the gap, two team members must attach the ropes to the hula hoop so that it can be suspended in the air at waist height. These two team members must then do their best to hold the hula hoop still in the air so that a teammate can be passed through it. Once the ropes are attached, the hula hoop cannot be touched by any team member.

The remaining team members must nominate at least one person to be passed through the gap. The gap cannot be stepped into or jumped through. The team member must not be touching the ground as they pass through the gap and the hula hoop must not be touched – and only the people holding the rope can touch the rope. Team members can be stationed on either side of the gap in the fence, but once they have chosen a side they cannot swap sides – unless they are passed through the gap.

### Discussion points
- What was the most difficult part of this challenge? Was it what you expected to be the trickiest part?
- If you didn't succeed the first time you tried, were you able to learn from your mistakes?
- How did it feel to be the person passed through the gap? Did you trust your teammates not to drop you?

### Expert challenge
- Can you complete the challenge without speaking?
- The two teammates suspending the hoop in the air must be replaced by two other teammates *during* the exercise, i.e. when someone else is passing through the gap. Can you keep the hoop still while you hand over the ropes to the next team member?

## 5. THE INVISIBLE MAZE

**Objective:** To find the invisible path through the maze.

*You will need*:

- Masking tape or chalk
- A whistle

*Suggested time limit*: 20 minutes
*Suggested team size*: 3–6

### Instructions

One team member becomes the guide, and they must direct their team through an invisible maze that only they can see the solution to. However, they can do this only by blowing a whistle as described on page 115 – they cannot say anything, and they cannot make any gestures or communicate in any other way.

Make sure none of the other team members can see the solution in advance, then start by using the masking tape or chalk to mark out a 3×3 grid on the floor, to create a larger version of the smallest example grid on page 116, making sure that there's enough room for a team member to stand in one square without being in another too. They should also be able to step from the middle of one square to the middle of a square next to it.

The guide points out where the starting square is, and then another team member is chosen to be the first explorer and must stand in the middle of it. The explorer then takes one step into a square of their choice next to the one they are in, moving only horizontally or vertically (not diagonally). Their aim is to discover the path shown on one of the example maps of your choosing on page 116.

If the explorer steps into the correct square (i.e. that which follows the path on the map), nothing happens and they are free to take another step to try and find the next square. If, however, they step into a square that isn't next on the path, the whistle is blown, and they must leave the maze. The next person now starts at the beginning of the maze, and the process begins again. Once everyone (other than the describer) has had a go, rotate around to the first person again and continue. Each explorer should use their memory to remember the part of the route successfully discovered so far, and not repeat the mistake the previous person made. Over several goes, the team will therefore discover the correct path.

Only one team member can be standing in the maze at any one point. The challenge is complete once the team find their way to the final square of the maze path.

### Discussion points

- How many times did you have to start again from the beginning of the maze? If you try again, can you do better?
- How did you decide which direction to try moving in when you were exploring the maze?
- Did you pay the same amount of attention when you were in the maze as when you were waiting for your turn? If not, how did that affect the team's ability to get through the maze?
- How did it feel when the whistle was blown, but no verbal feedback was given?
- If you completed the maze in silence, how did it change the way you worked as a team?

## Expert challenges

- Can you still complete the challenge if the explorer team members are not allowed to speak to one another? This means each member will need to remember the route on their own.
- Add more squares to create a more complex maze. You can easily have the guide design their own mazes.
- The guide could allow the path to cross over itself, but they would need to alert the team to this possibility.

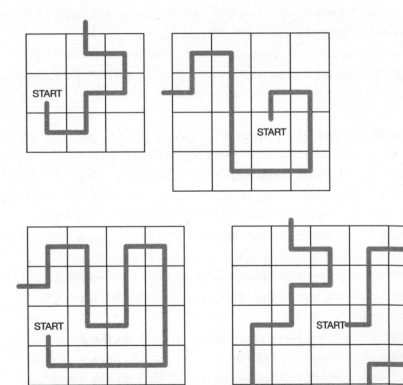

# LEADERLESS TASKS

## 1. LOWER LEVELS

**Objective:** To lower a hula hoop to the ground as a team.

*You will need*:

- A plastic hula hoop

*Suggested time limit:* 1 minute
*Suggested team size:* 6

**Instructions**

You and your team must lower a single plastic hula hoop to the ground.

Start with the team positioned around a hula hoop so that you are equally spread out. Hold the hoop so that it is level at about mid-chest height of the tallest team member. Then everyone should take a step back so that your arms are extended.

You must now each place the index finger of the hand you write with underneath the hoop, so that everyone is taking some of the weight of the hoop. The hoop cannot be touched by anything else.

When you are ready, start to lower the hoop to the ground as a group. If any member of the team breaks their contact with the hoop at any point, you must raise the hoop to the level you started at and begin again. When you reach the ground, the whole of the hoop must touch the ground at the same time – and on the way down, the hoop must be kept horizontal at all times.

The challenge is complete when the team successfully places the hoop on the ground, without having tilted it or anyone having broken contact with the hoop.

This challenge might sound easy, but it could prove deceptively difficult.

### Discussion points

- Was the challenge easier or harder than you expected it to be?
- Do you think it would be harder to raise or lower the hoop as a team in this way? Why? Test your theory.
- What happened when someone broke contact with the hoop? Did the challenge become easier after a restart, or more difficult?

### Expert challenge

- Can you complete the challenge again, but without speaking?
- Repeat the challenge. Everyone in the team must now use the index finger on the opposite hand to the one they used in the first attempt – i.e. the one they *don't* write with (unless they are ambidextrous). What difference do you notice?
- Is it still possible to complete the challenge if the whole team has their eyes closed?

## 2. PAPER TOWERS

**Objective:** To build the tallest tower you can using just two sheets of paper.

*You will need*:

- Four sheets of A4 paper
- Two pairs of scissors
- Two rolls of sticky tape
- A pencil, for testing

*Suggested time limit*: 15 minutes
*Suggested team size*: 4

**Instructions**
Split into two teams. Each team's task is to build a free-standing paper tower, using only two sheets of A4 paper each. They also have scissors and sticky tape. When the tower is finished, each team must be able to balance a standard pencil on top of the tower for 10 seconds to pass the challenge.

There is no limit to the amount of sticky tape you can use, but you are not permitted to use more than two sheets of paper per team, even if you damage or discard some of your paper during the construction.

After 15 minutes, place the two towers side by side. Each tower must be able to stand up on its own without any need for extra support. There must also be a place to balance a pencil on top of the tower when fully constructed, in order to test the tower's structural integrity. The pencil must stay in place for 10 seconds for the challenge to be complete. If you build the taller tower, but your tower cannot withstand the weight of the pencil, your team has not passed.

### Discussion points

- What would you do differently if you repeated the challenge? Were there any chances to make these changes during the first attempt?
- Did you waste any paper? Were you able to re-use it?
- Did anyone take the lead in this challenge? Was that helpful, or not?
- Did you make a plan before you started to build your tower? If yes, did your construction go according to plan? If you didn't, how would making a plan have changed the outcome?

### Expert challenge

- Can you complete the challenge without speaking?
- Repeat the challenge, but without using scissors or tape. You may not substitute these with any other materials. What is now the most difficult problem to overcome?
- Complete the construction in a relay. Divide the 15 minutes between the number of people in your team; so, for example, if there are five people in your team, you each have a three-minute time slot. The first person in the team constructs as much of the tower as possible in three minutes, and then hands their work over to the next team member. This continues until the 15 minutes are up and everyone in the team has spent some time constructing the tower. Teammates should not talk to each other during the exercise, so it is up to each team member to interpret the previous teammate's plan for the tower. How does this change the construction process?

# 3. THE HUMAN KNOT

**Objective:** To untangle linked arms until the team is standing in a circle.

*There are no extra materials required for this challenge.*

*Suggested time limit*: 15 minutes
*Suggested team size*: 6–8 people

## Instructions

You must untangle yourselves as a group from a 'human knot' made by linking arms, until you are standing in a circle.

Stand in a circle and take a step inwards so that you are standing shoulder to shoulder with your teammates. You should not be standing more than an arm's length away from any teammate. Each person must reach out and take the hand of someone across the circle. When everyone has hold of a hand, reach out and find another hand to hold, making sure you're not holding two hands that belong to the same person. You are now a human knot.

Slowly (and being careful of any arm-twisting), see if you can untangle your human knot as a group such that, when you are finished, you are once again standing in a circle. You may need to duck below and climb over other pairs of hands. You may also need to pass through loops made by pairs of arms linking together. You must not let go of the two hands you are holding, but you can readjust your grip to stop any arms from twisting and prevent injury.

Be sure to take your time, irrespective of the time limit, so as not to hurt either yourself or your teammates.

### Discussion points

- How did your expectations of the challenge affect the way you completed it?
- Did anyone take the lead in this challenge, and was that helpful for the group? If nobody took the lead, how would having a nominated leader have affected the challenge?
- Were there any unexpected results? If yes, what were they?

### Expert challenge

Can you untangle the human knot without speaking? How does it affect the speed with which you can safely complete the challenge?

## 4. TYRE TOWER

**Objective:** To move the tyres from left to right, ending in the same formation as at the start.

*You will need:*

- Four tyres – or bulky, stackable objects that are best lifted by multiple people
- Three free-standing vertical poles, arranged in a row – or something on the ground, to mark where the poles should go

*Suggested time limit*: 20 minutes
*Suggested team size*: 4–6

**Instructions**

This challenge is based on the classic 'Tower of Hanoi' challenge. Your aim is to move all of the tyres from one end of the line of poles to the other, following a strict set of rules. At the end of the challenge, the tyres must be stacked in the same formation as the one they started in.

Space out the three poles so that they are in a row, and place all four tyres over the pole on one end. Number the tyres from 1 to 4, with tyre 1 at the top of the stack and tyre 4 at the bottom. If your tyres are different sizes, place the smallest ones at the top of the stack.

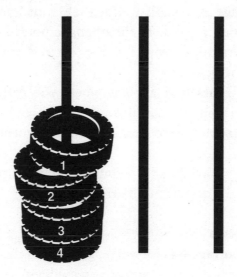

In order to complete the challenge, and transfer all the tyres from the left pole to the right pole, you must obey the following rules:

- Only one tyre can be moved at once
- You can only move the top tyre of any pile
- A tyre can never be placed above a tyre with a lower number. For example, tyre 1 can be put on top of tyre 3, but tyre 3 cannot be placed on tyre 1
- Tyres can be moved from any pole to any other pole, so long as the move obeys the rules above

The challenge is complete when all four tyres have been moved from the start pole to the opposite pole, and are stacked in the same formation, from 1 at the top to 4 at the bottom, as they were at the beginning.

If you find yourself at a point where you cannot make any progress, undo your steps until you find another way to proceed. You should try to avoid restarting the challenge from the beginning.

Warning: tyres are heavy, so you should take care and be sure to work carefully as a team on this task.

### Discussion points
- How important was forward planning to this exercise?
- If you reached a point where you could not make any more progress, how did you solve the problem?
- Was there a natural leader when you were completing the challenge? If yes, do you think they were helpful? Why? How did this affect the time taken to complete the challenge?

**Expert challenge**
- Add a fifth tyre. Can you still complete the challenge?
- Repeat the challenge, but without speaking to one another. If there was a leader before, does it now change? How can you communicate your ideas effectively and clearly, without talking?

# 5. GIANT'S FINGER

**Objective:** To lower a hula hoop over a pole, without touching either the hula hoop or the pole.

*You will need:*

- A hula hoop
- A free-standing vertical pole
- One 30 cm ruler per team member
- Plenty of space, so it is advisable to complete this challenge outside

*Suggested time limit*: 10 minutes
*Suggested team size*: 6

**Instructions**
Your team must raise a hula hoop from ground level and carry it over to a pole, which they must then lower the hoop over. The hoop may not be touched with anything except for the 30 cm rulers, and all team members must take equal responsibility for carrying the hoop.

Start by placing the hoop 5 metres away from the vertical pole. Team members must then position themselves around the hoop so that they can lift it into the air using the rulers. If the hoop is dropped at any point, the team must begin again from the starting point. Equally, if any team member's ruler breaks contact with the hoop, the challenge must be started again.

Once the hoop has been lifted and carried over to the vertical pole, the team must raise it over the top of the pole and lower it down with the pole in the middle. The hoop must be lowered gently, with all rulers touching it at all times. It cannot be dropped onto the ground.

The challenge is complete when the hoop has been lowered successfully over the pole and is sitting on the ground.

### Discussion points

- Which was harder – carrying the hoop over to the pole, or lowering it down?
- Were you able to use any other skills that you have gained in previous challenges to help you with this one?
- If contact was broken with the hoop at any point, how did the group adapt when restarting?

### Expert challenge

- Can you complete the challenge in the same amount of time if you are only able to use one hand to hold the ruler?
- Can you complete the challenge without talking to one another? How does that alter the difficulty of the challenge?
- You could try using a tyre instead of the hula hoop, but you will need to use sturdy poles instead of rulers to lift the tyre – such as broom handles.

# 6. PERFECT SQUARE

**Objective:** To create a perfect square with a loop of string.

*You will need*:

- A 5-metre-long piece of string, tied to make a loop

*Suggested time limit*: 10 minutes
*Suggested team size*: 6

## Instructions

Your team must – with their eyes closed – manipulate a loop of string from a circle into a square.

Start by standing in a circle and holding the string at waist height. Make sure the team is spread out evenly and that each member holds the string with both hands to ensure the loop is as close to a perfect circle as possible. Next, lower the string to the ground as a team, so that the whole circle of string touches the floor at the same time.

Everyone now closes their eyes, and takes a step back. Count to 10 as a group; then everyone takes a step forward and attempts to pick up the circle of string again. Now, all still with your eyes closed, bring the string back up to waist height and attempt to stand – as a team – so that you are holding the loop in such a way that it forms a perfect square.

When you think you have created the perfect square, lower the string back to the floor – still in the square shape – and let go. Take a step back and open your eyes.

Did you succeed? How close to a square is the shape you've created?

### Discussion points

- How easy was it to pick up the string again when you had taken a step back?
- Was there anything about the shape you formed that you were not expecting?
- What effect does everyone's eyes being closed have on the group?

### Expert challenge

- Can you still make the perfect square without speaking to each other after closing your eyes? You can speak and make a plan before starting, however.
- Are you still able to complete the challenge if you are not able to move your feet once you have taken the step forward to pick up the string again?
- Repeat the challenge but try to create a different regular-sided shape. Don't choose a shape that fits easily with the number of people in the group. For example, a team of six shouldn't attempt a hexagon, but could attempt a triangle.

## 7. OUT OF BOUNDS

**Objective:** To retrieve a bucket from inside a no-go zone using only ropes.

*You will need*:

- Six plastic cups
- A bucket
- One litre of water
- Two ropes, ideally each 2 metres long (skipping ropes will do)

*Suggested time limit*: 15 minutes
*Suggested team size*: 4

## Instructions

You must remove a bucket of hazardous material from inside a no-go zone, without spilling any of the contents. The only materials you may use to remove the bucket are two ropes, and no team members are allowed to touch the bucket directly.

Place the bucket on the floor and pour the litre of water into it. Space the cups evenly in a circle around the bucket, with each cup being 75 cm from the bucket. This is your out-of-bounds perimeter. Team members cannot step into the no-go zone and should avoid leaning into the area above the perimeter. (If the cups blow away, use some extra water to weigh them down.)

The team must now lift the bucket out of the perimeter to an empty space, and set it down safely on the ground. The bucket cannot be dragged outside of the no-go zone – it must be lifted into the air and only put down again once outside the zone.

If any of the liquid is spilled, the team must replace the bucket in the centre of the perimeter, pour in more water to bring it back to its original level, and start again.

The challenge is complete when the bucket is safely placed down outside the no-go zone without any water having being spilled.

## Discussion points
- Did you spill any water from the bucket? If yes, what did you do as a team to prevent this happening again?
- Was there a natural leader in the group? If yes, did it help your progress as a team to have a leader?
- Did you learn anything though trial and error? If yes, how did the process eventually help you to succeed?

### Expert challenge

- Move the cups so that they are 1.5 metres away from the bucket, and use 3.5-metre or longer ropes. Can you still retrieve the bucket?
- Fill the bucket so that it is half full. What effect does this have on the way you need to lift the bucket?

*Hint: Place the ropes either side of the bucket and twist them to create tension – you should be able to pick up the bucket when they are at the right tension. Be careful, since too much tension will spin the bucket and spill the liquid.*

# CHAPTER 4

# [SURVIVAL]

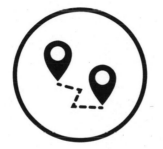

# SURVIVAL SKILLS

The battlefield is perhaps the most extreme environment in which human beings operate. In addition to coping with the lethal effects of high explosives, projectiles and chemicals, soldiers have to be able to eat, administer their needs and sleep. While survival in this context is difficult, it is by no means the only habitat in which soldiers may be called upon to exist in the course of their duties.

Increasingly, warfare is conducted without traditional front lines. This lack of definition, together with the widespread use of vulnerable aircraft over enemy-occupied territory, creates opportunities for soldiers to become isolated, requiring them to have a working knowledge of the skills necessary to survive. These techniques allow a soldier to navigate, find or build shelter, collect and purify water, hunt and forage for food, and use fire for warmth and cooking.

While Special Forces soldiers receive considerable training in survival skills across a wide range of environments, including jungles and deserts, all soldiers receive regular detailed revision and instruction in land navigation and the skills necessary to Survive, Evade, Resist and Extract. Training is enhanced for those whose duties risk bringing them into a survival situation (for example, aircrew), often building on the lessons learned by those who were forced to survive and evade in the Second World War.

Survival is much more difficult than it might immediately seem. Even in the temperate climate of the UK, cold and heat, precipitation and injury can threaten the survival of even the fittest individual in only a very few days. The primary consideration of any fugitive hoping to survive and evade must be the maintenance of good health; to this end, soldiers are trained in First Aid. Next, they must be able to use the environment to create shelter to stay out of the wind and rain, creating a base of operations to allow them to plan and preserve their faculties. Water, food and fire are the final priorities of those seeking to survive.

Life in any arduous environment is potentially precarious. The army gives its soldiers the skills to be resilient and to thrive in most conditions; while the chances of most soldiers experiencing a situation in which they would have to test these skills are low, it is important that they are practised and ready at all times. In this chapter, we will examine some of the ways in which a soldier might call upon their training to overcome the problems and hardships of their situation.

# SPEED PUZZLES

The ability to think quickly is a critical survival skill, so try the puzzles in this section and find out how *you* respond under pressure. There are two types of word puzzle, two types of number puzzle and two types of logic puzzle, so you can test a range of mental skills.

For each of the following exercises, time yourself and make a note of how long you took to solve each puzzle. A target time is given for each. Can you beat them all?

## WORD CIRCLE 1

Rearrange the letters in this circle to find as many words as you can. Every word must use the centre letter, plus two or more other letters – but you cannot use any individual letter more than once in a single word. There is one word that uses every letter.

Can you find 30 words in five minutes? There are over 60 to be found.

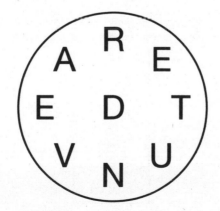

## WORD CIRCLE 2

Now try this second word circle puzzle. This time your target is to find 25 words in five minutes. There are over 50 to be found.

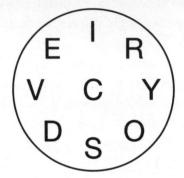

## WORD LADDER 1

Can you descend this ladder, one word at a time, to step from ARMY to BEDS? At each step you can change a single letter, but you can't rearrange the letters – and every step must contain a normal English word. For example, you could change CAT to COT to DOT to DOG, if you had a four-step ladder.

Can you solve it in less than two minutes?

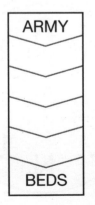

## WORD LADDER 2

Now try this second ladder. Can you solve it in less than one minute?

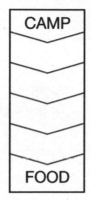

## NUMBER PYRAMID 1

Write a number in each empty block so that every block contains a value equal to the sum of the two blocks immediately beneath it.

Can you complete the entire pyramid in less than two minutes?

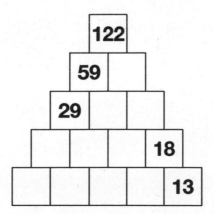

## NUMBER PYRAMID 2

Write a number in each empty block so that every block contains a value equal to the sum of the two blocks immediately beneath it.

Can you complete the entire pyramid in less than a minute?

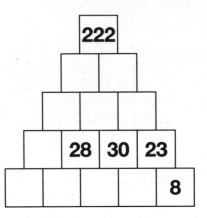

## BRAIN CHAIN 1

Can you solve this brain chain entirely in your head, without making any written notes? Start with the number at the left of each chain, then follow the arrows and apply each operation in turn. What number results?

Can you solve the brain chain, in your head, in less than a minute?

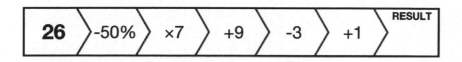

| 26 | -50% | ×7 | +9 | -3 | +1 | RESULT |

## BRAIN CHAIN 2

Try this second brain chain. Can you solve it, in your head, in less than 30 seconds?

| 19 | ×2 | -8 | $\times \frac{2}{3}$ | +60 | -10% | RESULT |

## NO FOUR IN A ROW 1

Write an 'X' or an 'O' in every empty square, so that no rows, columns or diagonals of four or more consecutive 'X's or 'O's are formed. Can you complete the entire puzzle in less than five minutes?

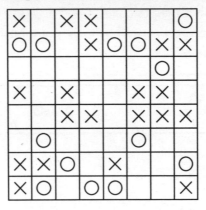

## NO FOUR IN A ROW 2

Again, write an 'X' or an 'O' in every empty square, so that no rows, columns or diagonals of four or more consecutive 'X's or 'O's are formed.

Can you complete this entire puzzle in less than three minutes?

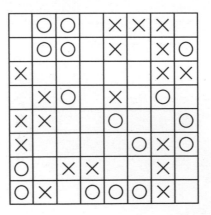

## DOMINOES 1

Draw along the dashed lines to divide the grid up into a complete set of dominoes, where a '0' represents a blank on a normal domino. You can use the check-off chart to keep track of which dominoes you've already placed. One is already marked for you, to get you started.

Can you place all the dominoes in less than ten minutes?

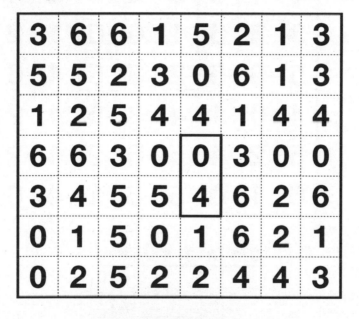

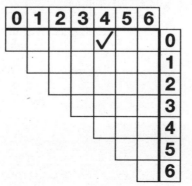

## DOMINOES 2

Now try this second dominoes puzzle. Can you place all the dominoes in less than seven minutes?

| 2 | 2 | 0 | 0 | 6 | 3 | 3 | 1 |
|---|---|---|---|---|---|---|---|
| 1 | 1 | 0 | 0 | 6 | 3 | 5 | 4 |
| 3 | 3 | 6 | 1 | 6 | 0 | 1 | 2 |
| 5 | 6 | 5 | 2 | 3 | 5 | 4 | 6 |
| 4 | 0 | 1 | 4 | 3 | 5 | 4 | 2 |
| 5 | 2 | 4 | 5 | 6 | 2 | 4 | 2 |
| 6 | 1 | 0 | 5 | 3 | 1 | 4 | 0 |

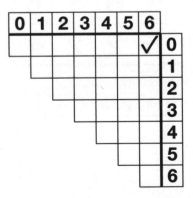

# CODE-BREAKING PUZZLES

Military information can be extremely sensitive, and transmitting information about location or enemy intelligence can put soldiers at risk. Codes are therefore useful for communicating in a secure way.

There are an infinite number of possible codes, ranging from the very simple to the very complex. These include mathematical codes based on prime numbers, and complex encoding schemes such as those created by the Enigma machine during the Second World War.

In this section, you will find a number of different codes to break, each revealing messages that a member of the army might encounter in their career.

## 1. MORSE CODE

Morse code was invented as a method of communicating messages using electrical pulses transmitted along telegraph wires. Each letter is made up of a pattern of dots and dashes, which can also be transmitted as short or long bleeps on a radio. They can also be represented by flashes of light of different length, or indeed in many other ways.

This is the Morse code alphabet:

# Morse Code

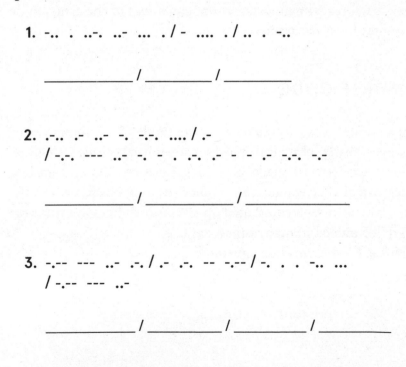

| | | | | | | | | | |
|---|---|---|---|---|---|---|---|---|---|
| A | •— | F | ••—• | K | —•— | P | •——• | U | ••— |
| B | —••• | G | ——• | L | •—•• | Q | ——•— | V | •••— |
| C | —•—• | H | •••• | M | —— | R | •—• | W | •—— |
| D | —•• | I | •• | N | —• | S | ••• | X | —••— |
| E | • | J | •——— | O | ——— | T | — | Y | —•—— |
| | | | | | | | | Z | ——•• |

Here are three phrases, written out in Morse code.

Use the table to work out what the messages are. Each word is separated by a forward slash (/). Write your decoded text in the spaces shown.

1. —•• • ••—• ••— ••• • / — •••• • / •• • —••

   _____ / _____ / _____

2. •—•• •— ••— —• —•— •••• / •—
   / —•—• ——— ••— —• — •—• • — — — •— —• —• ——

   _____ / _____ / _____

3. —•—— ——— ••— —• / •— —• —— —•—— / —• • • —•• •••
   / —•—— ——— ••—

   _____ / _____ / _____ / _____

Now try the same with these three further phrases, where the dots and dashes are represented by words:

Dash dot dot dot, dot, / dash, dot dot dot dot, dot /
dash dot dot dot, dot, dot dot dot, dash

_____ / _____ / _____

Dash dot dash dot, dot dash dot, dot dot, dash, dot dot,
dash dot dash dot, dot dash, dot dash dot dot / dash,
dot, dot dash dot, dot dash dot, dot dash, dot dot, dash
dot

_____ / _____

Dot dash dash dot, dot dash dot, dash dash dash, dash,
dot, dash dot dash dot, dash / dash, dot dot dot dot,
dot / dash dot, dot dash, dash, dot dot, dash dash dash,
dash dot

_____ / _____ / _____

## 2. SEMAPHORE

Over the years, people in the military have needed to convey information over long distances, particularly at sea. One such historical system was semaphore. Although the modern army no longer uses it, it was, for example, employed during the Boer War and in the First World War trenches.

Semaphore uses a system of two flags held up at different angles to represent different letters of the alphabet.

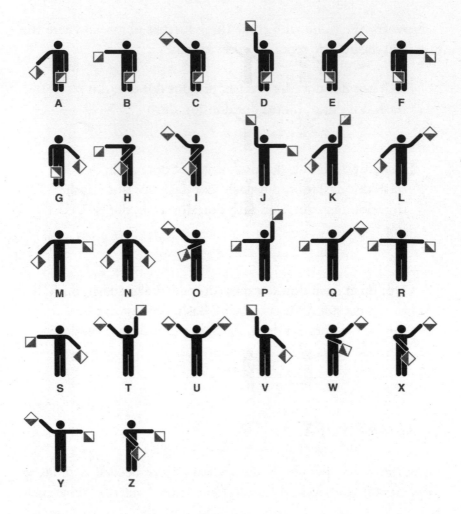

To represent a space, point both flags straight downwards.

Here are three messages that have been delivered in semaphore. Can you decipher them?

**1.**

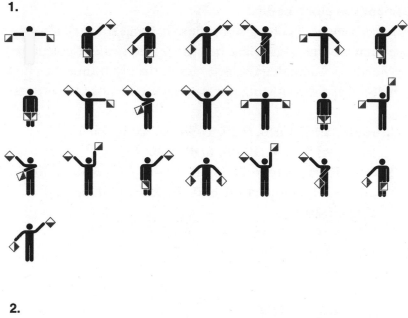

**2.**

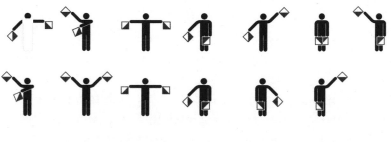

**3.**

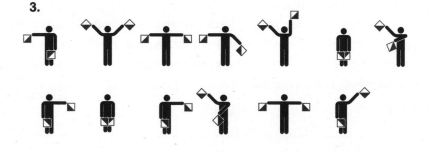

### Semaphore clock codes

Another way of encoding semaphore is using clock times, where you imagine the flags being held at the equivalent positions to the hands on an analogue clock face at the given time. See if you can decipher the following phrases represented by clock times:

1. 10:00, 9:15, 10:10, 9:20, 10:00, 6:30, 10:15, 10:45, 10:10, 9:15, 6:30, 10:00, 6:10, 6:40, 8:15
2. 8:10, 10:45, 6:40, 6:00, 6:30, 10:00, 7:45, 6:10, 6:30, 8:15, 6:40, 6:50, 7:45, 10:40, 7:20, 6:10, 6:30, 6:20, 10:10, 7:20
3. 9:20, 6:10, 7:20, 6:00, 6:30, 6:45, 6:40, 6:50, 8:00, 10:10, 9:00

# 3. CAESAR SHIFT

One of the oldest ways of encrypting messages is via the Caesar shift. It is named after Julius Caesar, who used it when he was writing important messages about military matters.

It is a simple substitution code in which each letter is replaced with a different letter from the alphabet, the alphabet having been shifted a certain number of places forwards or backwards, wrapping around from Z to A.

Here is an example of a Caesar shift cipher with a shift of three. Each letter in the top line is encoded as the letter in the bottom line. To read the message, you change each encoded letter in the bottom row back to its original unencoded letter in the top row.

| A | B | C | D | E | F | G | H | I | J | K | L | M | N | O | P | Q | R | S | T | U | V | W | X | Y | Z |
|---|---|---|---|---|---|---|---|---|---|---|---|---|---|---|---|---|---|---|---|---|---|---|---|---|---|
| D | E | F | G | H | I | J | K | L | M | N | O | P | Q | R | S | T | U | V | W | X | Y | Z | A | B | C |

Here are two phrases encoded using the exact substitution shown on the previous page. Can you decode them?

1. PHHW HYHUB FKDOOHQJH
2. FDOO WKH ERPE GLVSRVDO WHDP

For the following two phrases, the alphabet has been moved forward by between two and five letters. Can you work out the shifts and reveal the phrases?

3. GEPP XLI QENSV KIRIVEP
4. EQPVCEV, YCKV QWV

For these two codes, see if you can you work out the shifts without any hints. What do they decode to?

5. VLR'OB FK VLRO LTK QFJB KLT
6. OSVXUBOYKJ KDVRUYOBK JKBOIK

## 4. ATBASH

Atbash codes are alphabet based, just like Caesar shifts, and were originally designed to encode the Hebrew alphabet (thus the name, which is a contraction of two Hebrew letter names), although they can be used with any letter-based alphabet. They work by reversing the alphabet and substituting letters in the reversed order, so that A is represented by Z, B is represented by Y and so on, through to Z being represented by A, as shown in the table below.

| A | B | C | D | E | F | G | H | I | J | K | L | M | N | O | P | Q | R | S | T | U | V | W | X | Y | Z |
|---|---|---|---|---|---|---|---|---|---|---|---|---|---|---|---|---|---|---|---|---|---|---|---|---|---|
| Z | Y | X | W | V | U | T | S | R | Q | P | O | N | M | L | K | J | I | H | G | F | E | D | C | B | A |

Can you work out what the following messages say, by decoding using the Atbash cipher?

1. NRORGZIB LKVIZGRLMH
2. R'N KILNLGRMT BLF GL ORVFGVMZMG
3. GSRH KOZGLLM SZH GSRIGB HLOWRVIH
4. XLMTIZGFOZGRLMH, OZMXV XLIKLIZO
5. FHV GSV HGIVZN ZH XLEVI
6. DV ZIV FMWVI ZGGZXP

# 5. CODED LETTERS

## NATO codewords

If you have ever tried to spell your name to someone over the telephone, you will probably have discovered the challenges of dictating letters accurately. The NATO phonetic alphabet helps to solve this problem, as it is harder to mishear when each letter is assigned a distinct word. This is particularly useful in military communications where accuracy is crucial when communicating information.

Here is the complete list:

| A | Alpha | H | Hotel |
|---|---|---|---|
| B | Bravo | I | India |
| C | Charlie | J | Juliett |
| D | Delta | K | Kilo |
| E | Echo | L | Lima |
| F | Foxtrot | M | Mike |
| G | Golf | N | November |

| O | Oscar | U | Uniform |
|---|-------|---|---------|
| P | Papa | V | Victor |
| Q | Quebec | W | Whiskey |
| R | Romeo | X | X-Ray |
| S | Sierra | Y | Yankee |
| T | Tango | Z | Zulu |

These codenames can also be used more subtly to transfer information. For example, the letter below contains a secret message concealed using the NATO phonetic alphabet. Your challenge is to read the letter and work out what the message is:

*Ms Caroline Scott*
*37 Pipe Road*
*Mumbai*
*India*

*Dear Mike,*
*I was very glad to receive your letter, I'm happy you are doing well and progressing so quickly. It sounds like Charlie is getting up to plenty of mischief, as usual! He always was something of an alpha male.*

*Papa is the same as ever, he went to the shops for washing powder today and came back with three aubergines and a new bin for the bathroom. We are starting a tango class on Monday, which should be a fun challenge. The uniform is very strict, I have to buy some special dancing shoes with high heels – I have found a brand called Romeo which seems quite good value.*

*Do you have any holiday plans? We are thinking of going to Echo Point in the north of the country for a long weekend – not quite the same as our usual trip to the Ganges Delta, but it should make a pleasant change.*

*All my love,*
*Caroline*

## A punctual letter

The following letter from an army captain has a word concealed within it using one of the codes already covered in this section. Can you crack the code to find the hidden word?

*Dear Major,*
*I am a Captain in the Royal Engineers posted in Brunei. I am writing to inform you of our progress on the training exercises we have been assigned – so far everything is going well.*

*The troops are in good spirits and are supporting each other well. The only problem we have encountered is fatigue in the difficult conditions.*

*Exercises in the jungle naturally bring some challenges and some soldiers have been badly bitten by insects. Mosquitos in particular are proving a nuisance. We are running low on medication to treat these wounds – some more supplies would be greatly appreciated.*

*We have completed half of the training exercises and some of the new recruits show great promise. Particularly our latest addition from Sandhurst – Max. His ingenuity in the field is second to none.*

*I hope all is going well in your regiment.*
*I will be sending further updates once we have completed the remainder of the exercises. If you have any news about*

*the supplies, please let myself and my medical team know.*
*I look forward to hearing from you.*

*Regards,*
*Mark*

## Letter code

This letter between two friends has an important word concealed within it, using a code that has been covered earlier in this chapter. Can you crack the code and reveal the secret word?

*Dear Dottie,*

*It was wonderful to receive your last letter; it sounds like the cicadas have come out in full force! Your anecdotes always give us a good laugh.*

*We have just got back to base after a four-day-long training exercise and proper beds are proving a much-needed antidote.*

*We haven't seen a great deal of wildlife while we have been out here, but yesterday that all changed very suddenly. A huge anaconda shot out of the undergrowth onto the path and we had to dash out of the way. Thankfully it seemed to have its eyes fixed on something to eat already.*

*Training is challenging as ever, our new sergeant likes to make sure we have dotted all our 'i's and crossed our 't's. I do tend to get up around an hour early to clean my kit and make sure everything is in order.*

*As part of our schedule, we have watched other regiments nearby doing their exercises – it's quite an experience seeing how other sergeants and new recruits operate.*

*It would be lovely to organise a visit soon; I know we discussed a few dates but I have checked other times and there seems to be a good selection. We all have a lot to do this week, but hopefully after next Monday it won't be so much of a to-do to work something out.*

*All my love,*
*Jess*

## 6. NUMERICAL CODES

The British Army has several barracks around the UK where soldiers live and train. Below is a list of names of a few of these barracks. They have, however, been written in code, with the letters in each word being replaced by numbers. Can you figure out the code – without any help – to reveal the list of names?

**1.** 2-5-1-3-8-12-5-25
**2.** 18-1-7-12-1-14
**3.** 2-1-11-5-18
**4.** 12-15-14-4-5-19-2-15-18-15-21-7-8

These names have a different code:

**5.** 24-15-26-9-12
**6.** 9-12-2-26-15-0-26-9-7-18-15-15-22-9-2

And these final two barracks are encoded using a more complex code:

**7.** 2-8-05-18-20-16-04-18-02
**8.** 18-02-4-6-04-18-4

# 7. ANAGRAM PUZZLES

Please ignore any spaces and punctuation when solving these anagrams.

### A unit of confusion
The words below are all anagrams of unit sizes within the army.

They each also have one extra letter added to them, which when added together across all eight anagrams spell out a further unit size.

Can you unscramble the words, find the extra letters and reveal the hidden unit?

1. ABRIDGED
2. PORTUGAL BITE
3. VALIANT BOT
4. TIGER MINE
5. NOSY CAMP
6. IRON QUADS
7. NOT A LOOP
8. PROTON

## Unscramble the ranks

The following words are all ranks of officer and soldier in the British Army. Can you unscramble the words, and then sort them according to whether they are officer or soldier ranks?

1. AIR BRIDGE
2. A TIN CAP
3. NO CELLO
4. CAR OR LOP
5. ENLARGE
6. TUNE IN LATE
7. OR JAM
8. PAIR VET
9. STERN AGE
10. GENERATORS JAM
11. CRAFT FAIR OWNER

## Personal equipment

Each of these pieces of personal equipment has had the letters rearranged into alphabetical order. Can you unscramble them to reveal some of the equipment that a soldier in the army might carry with them?

1. GNU
2. ADIOR
3. ADEEGNR
4. EEHLMT
5. BDOY AMORRU
6. ABCMOT CGHILNOT

# ENIGMATIC PUZZLES

Stay sharp and stay alive. See if you can work out what's going on in the following puzzles, which require you to think cleverly to solve them.

## 1. ARMY UNITS

The British Army has a hierarchical command structure with multiple different regiments and corps. Each of these is composed of different numbers of soldiers and officers, who report to different people. Below is a list of units, but each one has been concealed. Delete one letter from each pair of letters to reveal the names of each unit.

You have already seen these units in the previous section, which may help.

> AD PI RV EI AS LI DO TN
> BA RB IL EG DA ED ES
> SB OA RT ET LA BL FI ON MN
> RP EA SG CI IM DE AN LT
> CH OA LM OP FA SN HY
> DS IQ LU SA ED NR IO SN
> LP SL EA IT DO RO NM
> PT IR SO EO PS

## 2. OFFICER RANKS

The following word fragments make up six army officer ranks, which you have also seen in the previous section. The fragments

157

have been organised in alphabetical order. Can you work out which fragment belongs to which rank?

| | | |
|---|---|---|
| AL | BRI | CAP |
| COL | EL | ER |
| GAD | GEN | IER |
| IN | JOR | LIE |
| MA | NA | NT |
| ON | TA | UTE |

## 3. BRITISH BEASTS

| Rule A | Rule B | Rules A and B | Neither A nor B |
|---|---|---|---|
| | | | |
| | | | |

The words in the list below either comply, or don't comply, with two underlying rules: A and B.

See if you can work out what the two core rules, A and B, are so that when you add the given words into the table there are exactly two per column. For example, rule A might be 'It shares its name with a household job'.

Car
Centurion
Challenger
Chaplin
Churchill
Cleaner
Cook
Cromwell

## 4. AN UNUSUAL OCCUPATION

The following words are all occupations that exist within the army, but they have had any of the letters found in the word 'army' removed from them. For example, 'march' would become 'ch', since the 'a', 'r' and 'm' would be removed.

Can you work out what each of the following occupations are?

Nuse
Bickle
Dog Hndle
Dive
Gudsn
ine
usicin
Office
Ptoope

## 5. AFRICAN DEPLOYMENTS

The British Army, at the time of writing, deploys troops in seven different African countries. These countries are listed below, but every other letter has been removed. Can you work out what the countries are?

S_U_H   _U_A_

S_M_L_A

D_M_C_A_I_   R_P_B_I_   O_   T_E   _O_G_

K_N_A

N_G_R_A

G_B_N

M_L_W_

# 6. A START IN THE ARMY

The expressions below all have their roots in military settings. Can you match them up to their modern meanings?

| Expression | Modern Meaning |
| --- | --- |
| Avant-garde | Very quickly |
| Balls to the wall | An unpredictable character |
| Bite the bullet | Unclaimed territory |
| Loose cannon | Endure strong criticism |
| No man's land | Novel and experimental |
| On the double | Deal with the inevitable displeasure |
| Take the flak | Complete a task with intense effort |

# 7. ANCIENT CIVILISATIONS

What connects the answers to the following clues?

- A person from the home city of Helen, Paris and Priam
- A Greek god who preceded the Olympians
- Wife of Jupiter
- A person from a famous rival of Athens in the south-eastern Peloponnese

# MEMORY TESTS

As you saw in some of the exercises in Chapter 3, paying attention to detail and remembering what you have seen can be a critical skill. It can make the difference between success or failure, or between survival and death.

Try the memory tasks in this section, to practise your skills. Don't worry if you struggle at first, since, as with all skills, it can take time and practice to improve at using your memory.

## 1. PRESENT AND CORRECT

When soldiers are taught how to navigate in the British Army, they learn how to use real-life landmarks on the ground to help them relate to the information shown on the map and establish their exact location. To do this, they are told to consider the following:

> DIRECTION
> DISTANCE
> CONVENTIONAL SIGNS
> RELIEF
> ALIGNMENT
> PROXIMITY
> SHAPE

Study this list for two minutes, paying close attention to the order that the above considerations are presented in.

When the time is up, cover up the list above and then number the list overleaf to show the order in which the features were initially presented, using 1 to indicate the feature that came first, and 7 to indicate the last.

ALIGNMENT
CONVENTIONAL SIGNS
DIRECTION
DISTANCE
PROXIMITY
RELIEF
SHAPE

Check back to see how you did.


## 2. MEMORY DECK

- For this challenge you will need two people, and one pack of standard playing cards

*Suggested time limit:* 20 minutes

This challenge is a more complex version of a 'memory matching pairs' game. Start by splitting the deck into one pile of red cards and one pile of black cards. Take one pile each.

You and the other person must spread out the playing cards from half of the pack face-down in front of you. Make sure you are back to back and cannot see the other person's cards. Now take turns, turning over the cards one by one, and call out the card you have uncovered to your teammate. After every call from your teammate, you have the opportunity to turn over a card and see if the number value matches.

For example, if your teammate turns over an eight, you can turn one card over and see if it is also an eight. If they match, you each turn the cards face up. If not, both cards are replaced face-down. It's then your go to turn over a new card and call it out. The challenge is complete when all cards from both piles have been matched successfully.

## 3. NUMBERS AND CHUNKS

Read the following number for 30 seconds and try to memorise it:

09869846

Then, after the 30 seconds, write the number sequence down on a separate piece of paper.

How well could you remember it? Check your answer.

Now repeat the exercise with each of the following numbers in turn:

175697456
2827487657
35718401735

Did you find it harder as the numbers became longer? To help remember longer number strings, like the ones above, you can use a technique known as 'chunking'. Instead of trying to remember a long sequence of separate digits, group them into more meaningful chunks. In this way, you reduce the number of elements that you need to remember.

For example, the number 50187472 could be split into 50 18 747 2, so you can now remember it as 'fifty', 'adult', 'jumbo', 'two' – or some other sequence that makes sense to you. In this case 'adult' refers to the age of becoming an adult at 18, and 'jumbo' refers to the 747 jumbo jet. Coming up with these might take you some time, but it's easier to remember these four items than eight separate digits.

You can also simply group the numbers into larger numbers, remembering 50187472 as 50, 18, 74, 72, in a similar way to how you might break up a phone number.

Now you have learned about chunking, try the memory exercise again – but give yourself 60 seconds per number to give you some time to practise chunking it. Can you use this method to remember longer numbers more efficiently?

94859485
01747603
820571232
4246720535

## 4. ALL CHANGE?

Cover over the opposite page, then give yourself two minutes to study the set of graticules below.

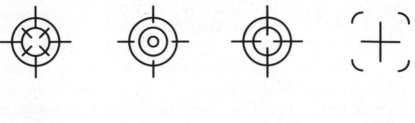

When you've finished, cover the left-hand page and look at the images below. The images have changed places and four have been swapped for new images. Can you spot the new images without looking back at the left-hand page?

## 5. SLEEP TEST

It's crucial to remain vigilant and constantly absorbing information so that, when an unexpected situation occurs, you are ready with the details you need.

Take five minutes to read the passage below. When you have finished reading, cover it up and try to answer the questions about the text on the following page. The questions will cover both the content and structure of the passage, so pay careful attention.

SLEEP:

- Sleep is a fundamental component of physical recovery
- It is important to establish a bedtime routine for effective sleep
- During periods of sleep restriction, naps should be taken where possible to minimise sleep debt

TARGETS:

- Seven to eight hours of sleep in every 24-hour period
- For most effective sleep, go caffeine and alcohol free for six hours before sleep
- You should not use electronic devices for one hour before sleep

## Questions

1. How many hours of sleep should you aim for in a 24-hour period?
2. How long before sleep should you switch off electronic devices?
3. How many bullet points were under the heading 'Targets'?
4. How many times does the word 'sleep' appear in the passage?
5. What should you avoid doing in the six hours before you sleep?

## 6. FOLLOW THE DIFFERENCE

You have five minutes to read and remember the passage below.

    After the five minutes is over, cover up this passage and read the text on the page opposite. Can you spot *ten* differences between the first passage and the second, without looking back to the first?

*When you reach the footbridge, cross directly over the river and continue north at a steady pace. In 30 km you'll reach a steep incline with a bridleway in front of you. Cross the bridleway (remember to look out for horses!) and follow the footpath up the steep hill. Be careful – once you reach the top there's a steep drop on the eastern side. Nice spot for a picnic! Sun will set at around 2000 hrs on Wednesday, so as long as you've got good visibility, you'll have plenty of daylight left when the trek is over. Remember to close the gates behind you.*

*When you reach the footpath, cross directly over the stream and continue north at a steady rate. In 30 km you'll reach a sharp incline with a bridleway in front of you. Cross the bridleway (remember to look out for horses!) and follow the footpath up the steep hill. Be careful – once you reach the top there's a steep drop on the eastern side. Sun will rise at around 2000 hrs on Wednesday so as long as you've got great visibility, you'll have plenty of time left when the hike is over. Remember to open the gates behind you.*

## 7. CURRENT DEPLOYMENTS

The map overleaf shows some of the locations where British Army forces are actively operating around the world.

You have two minutes to study this map. When the time is up, cover the page and see if you can fill in the map in the same way on the opposite page. When you're done, check your answers. Did you remember them all?

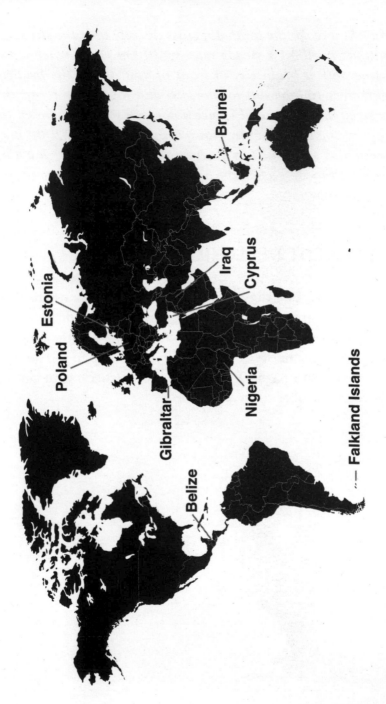

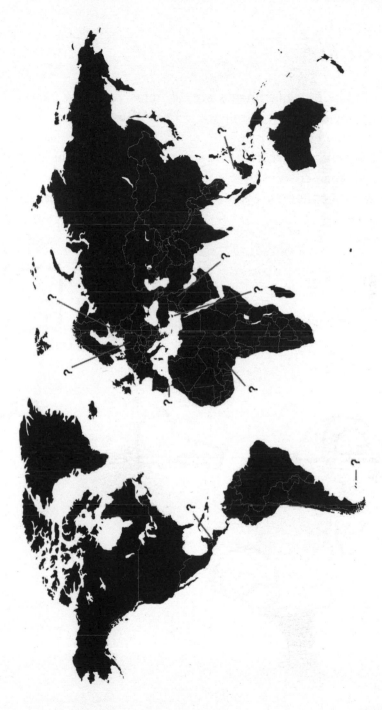

## 8. KIT BAG

The following eight images are all items you have packed into your kitbag. When you unpack it after an expedition, you notice one of the items is missing.

Study this page carefully and try to memorise the items you packed, then cover it over. On the opposite page, you will see a word list of the items you returned with. Which item has gone missing?

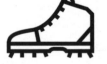

SLEEPING BAG
ROPE
MAP
WATERPROOF JACKET
BOOTS
TENT
HELMET

## 9. FLOOR PLANS

The image below shows a floor plan of one of the buildings in your training compound. Each room has at least one item in it that you need to remember the location of. Study it for two minutes, then turn over the page and see if you can fill in the blank floor plan overleaf, marking where each item was.

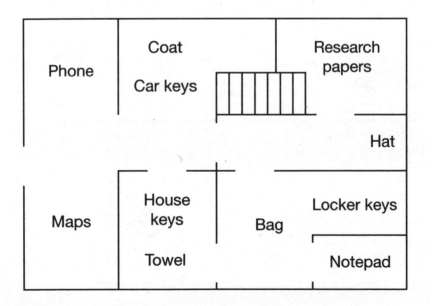

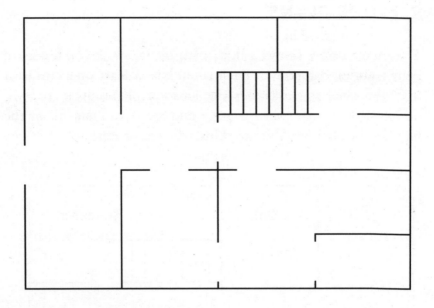

# 10. GRID MEMORY

The following question will require some knowledge from Chapter 1 concerning four-figure grid references. If you haven't completed that challenge yet, go back to it and revisit this question afterwards to test your skills.

Now, can you memorise the following four-digit grid references, and then use them to shade in an image on the grid overleaf? Each reference indicates one square on the grid that needs to be shaded in.

Give yourself a few minutes to memorise the grid references, then turn over the page and try to fill in the grid. You'll know if you have remembered them correctly when you shade them in.

| | | | |
|---|---|---|---|
| 3415 | 3514 | 3613 | 3714 |
| 3815 | 3916 | 4017 | 4118 |

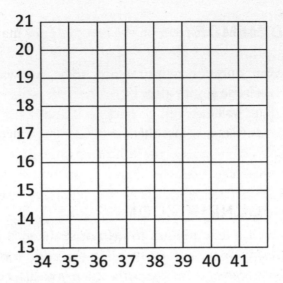

## 11. FIT AS A FIDDLE

Spend up to five minutes memorising the following fitness itinerary. After the five minutes is up, cover up the itinerary and answer the questions opposite. Pay close attention to the order in which the exercises are presented.

Thirty sit-ups
Twenty press-ups
Fifteen burpees
Ten squats
Twenty-five press-ups
A 15-minute jog

**Questions**

1. What was the first item on the list, and how many were required?
2. How many press-ups were on the list?
3. What exercise comes after burpees?
4. How long was the jog?
5. How many stages were there to the fitness itinerary in total?

## 12. CONFOUNDING COMPOUND

The grid below is a basic map of a compound you will be required to navigate on the ground from memory. For security, you cannot take a map of the compound with you. Each of the shaded areas represents a building.

Study the grid for five minutes, and then turn over the page. Can you re-create the pattern – and therefore the map of the compound – on the empty grid? When you're done, check the original picture and see if you were correct.

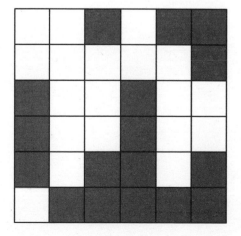

Now recall the pattern:

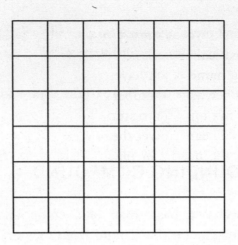

Check back. How did you do?

# 13. NAMES AND NUMBERS

This challenge asks you to use your memory skills and apply them to mathematical exercises.

The following names each have a number next to them, and you must remember which number is next to which name.

Give yourself five minutes to study the text, then turn over the page and, see if you can answer the simple maths questions overleaf, which use the names in place of numbers. Your answer should be given numerically.

Anne 1
Charles 2
Edward 8
Elizabeth 2
George 6
Henry 8
James 2
Mary 2
Richard 3
Victoria 1
William 4

**Questions**
1. Elizabeth x Richard = _____
2. Charles + Victoria = _____
3. George – William = _____
4. Edward – Henry = _____
5. What name is equal to the result of Anne + Victoria + James + Mary?

For a bonus, the people in this list all have something in common. What is it, and what do the numbers signify?

# 14. MEMORY MATHS

Study the grid below for a couple of minutes and pay close attention to the position of the numbers within the grid.

The following questions will then ask you to solve mathematical questions, but instead of numbers you will be shown a grid with the empty cells shaded in and instructions for the numbers that you have memorised in those squares.

The answers to the calculations will also be numbers that appear in the grid below. Mark your answers by placing an 'X' where you think the correct number appears.

Here is the grid to memorise:

| | | |
|---|---|---|
| 4 | 2 | 15 |
| 24 | 9 | 5 |
| 3 | 36 | 1 |

Now try these questions:

**1.**

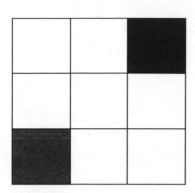

Dark grey ÷ light grey = ?

**2.**

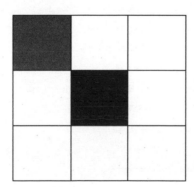

Dark grey × light grey = ?

**3.**

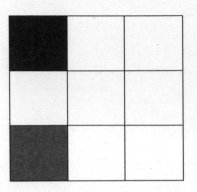

Dark grey - light grey = ?

**4.**

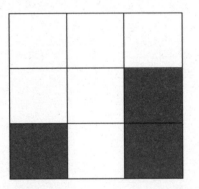

What is the total value of the shaded cells?

## 15. WORD ASSOCIATION

Spend a few minutes studying the words and pictures below.

Each word has been placed next to a piece of fruit. Memorise the pairings, and their locations on the page. Then, when you're ready, turn over the page and answer the questions.

**TANK**

**HELICOPTER**

**AMBULANCE**

**TRUCK**

**RADIO**

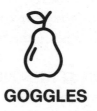
**GOGGLES**

**HELMET**

**MAP**

**BOOTS**

**Questions**

1. Which piece of fruit was paired with the helmet?
2. What piece of equipment was the melon paired with? Which two pieces of equipment were directly above, and directly to the left of it?
3. What word was the lemon paired with?
4. Which fruit was 'able to fly'?

## 16. CODES AND PASSWORDS

You have been given the following passwords and codes during an intelligence operation. Security measures prevent you from writing them down, in case they are picked up by enemy hands. Instead, you are given five minutes to memorise them, after which they will disappear.

Study the codes, then after five minutes cover them up. Can you fill in the blanks and gain access?

STAFF ENTRANCE: 3658
Central Database: O4N3Y2X1
Your Personal Codename: Falcon12
Access Code 4: 890Q4f
Emergency Shutdown: NAID44ISBO

Now fill in the blanks:

Access Code 4: _____
Central Database: _____
Emergency Shutdown: _____
STAFF ENTRANCE: _____
Your Personal Codename: _____

# 17. REMEMBER THIS RECIPE

You are an army chef in training, and you have been given the following recipe to attempt during a practice expedition.

Give yourself five minutes to study it closely and memorise as many details as possible. Then cover it up and read the instructions that follow. (Note that this is not a real recipe – it is only for the purposes of this exercise.)

Sausage Stew – serves 10

Ingredients
- 12 medium sausages
- 2 kg tomatoes
- 3 white onions
- 2 kg carrots
- 3 cans butter beans
- 4 red peppers
- Salt and pepper
- Oil

Method
1. Cover bottom of large pan in oil, and place on medium heat
2. Dice carrots and onions, and add to the oil. When both are soft but not browning, add sausages, chopped into four pieces each
3. After 2 mins, add red peppers (diced)
4. When the sausage pieces are thoroughly cooked, add tomatoes (quartered). Turn heat down

5. After 10 mins, add the butter beans. Stir. Simmer for 10 more mins
6. Add salt and pepper to taste. Ensure sausages are cooked through. Serve

You now arrive at camp and find a hungry group of solders awaiting their dinner. Can you remember the recipe? Answer the questions opposite to find out.

**Questions**
1. How many of the ingredients needed to be diced?
2. What quantity of tomatoes was needed?
3. What ingredient was added after sausages?
4. How many people does the recipe serve?
5. What is the last ingredient to be mentioned?
6. How long does the dish simmer for after the butter beans are added?

# 18. RECONNAISSANCE READY

You are infiltrating an unknown compound that you believe may be involved in poaching activity. Due to thick jungle overhead, it has not been possible to provide your team with an aerial photograph of the area. A previous reconnaissance mission has, however, managed to supply you with the verbal instructions overleaf. You have no more than ten minutes to memorise them.

Each square on your blank map overleaf represents roughly 100 metres on the ground, and gates are marked with an X. When you have finished memorising your instructions, cover them over and then mark your route in pencil, making a note of any sentry points. Which gate do you exit from?

*Avoid open courtyard areas. Enter the compound through the north gate, checking for sentries close to the gate in the building on your right. If there are none, proceed forward (due south) 300 metres until you reach the building directly in front of you.*

*There is a sentry point in the central section of the building south of the west gate, so your best route is to continue through the building directly in front of you for 200 metres until you exit on the south side of it.*

*Stay close to the wall. Turn 90 degrees anticlockwise and walk forward for 100 metres, then turn a further 90 degrees anticlockwise and walk forward for 100 metres. Now turn 90 degrees to your right and continue forward 200 metres. The structure to your left is low enough that you can climb over it. When you have done so, take the gate to your right.*

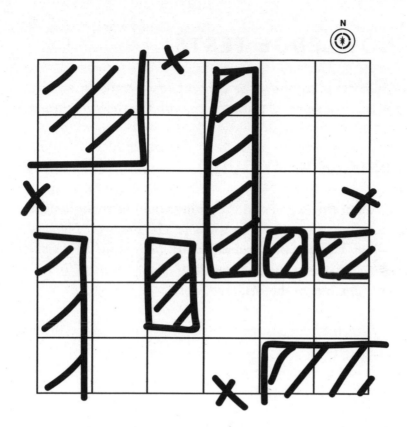

# KNOWLEDGE TESTS

It's important to know the context of operations, so test your knowledge of some relevant topics with the following quizzes.

## 1. BRITISH ARMY QUIZ

1. What title is given to the professional head of the British Army?
   a. Chief of the General Staff
   b. Chief of the Defence Staff
   c. Chief of the Military Staff

2. Which of these is the highest officer rank in the British Army?
   a. Lieutenant General
   b. Major General
   c. General

3. As of 2019, which of these countries is the British Army *not* currently operating in?
   a. Belize
   b. Bolivia
   c. Brunei

4. What does the acronym AOSB stand for?
   a. Army of Staff Brigade
   b. Army Officer Selection Board
   c. Army Outer Section Briefing

5. How many soldier ranks are there in the British Army?
   a. 5
   b. 6
   c. 7

6. What is the name given to the current camouflage pattern used for combat clothing in the British Army?
   a. Multi-terrain pattern (MTP)
   b. Maximum cover pattern (MCP)
   c. All fields pattern (AFP)

7. Where in the UK would you find Army Headquarters?
   a. Andover
   b. Bristol
   c. Cardiff

## 2. HISTORY OF THE BRITISH ARMY QUIZ

1. In what year was the Royal Military Academy Sandhurst founded?
   a. 1887
   b. 1927
   c. 1947

2. What is the name of the conflict between Argentina and the UK in 1982?
   a. South Islands War
   b. Falklands War
   c. Argentine War

3. In what year did conscription, also known as National Service, end?
   a. 1950
   b. 1960
   c. 1970

4. Which event in 1707 led to the first use of the term 'British Army'?
   a. The union of England and Scotland
   b. The Seven Years' War
   c. The Monmouth Rebellion

## 3. BRITISH MONARCHY QUIZ

1. Which member of the British royal family attended RMA Sandhurst from 2005 to 2006?
   a. Prince William
   b. Prince Harry
   c. Prince Andrew

2. Who is the Commander-in-Chief of the British Armed Forces?
   a. Queen Elizabeth II
   b. Prince Philip
   c. Prince Charles

3. Which of the following is *not* a Commonwealth Realm?
   a. Papua New Guinea
   b. Tuvalu
   c. Samoa

4. When the 1st Buckingham Palace Company was formed in 1937, what was its role?
    a. A decoy unit for intelligence operations
    b. A Girl Guide patrol
    c. A ceremonial military jazz band

# 4. UK GEOGRAPHY QUIZ

1. What is the name of the highest mountain in the UK?
    a. Ben Nevis
    b. Scafell Pike
    c. Snowdon

2. Which of these UK rivers is the longest?
    a. River Trent
    b. River Avon
    c. River Severn

3. How many ceremonial counties does England have?
    a. 24
    b. 36
    c. 48

4. How many national parks are there in the UK?
    a. 10
    b. 15
    c. 20

5. Approximately what percentage of the land area of Wales is a National Park?
    a. 10 per cent

b. 15 per cent

c. 20 per cent

6. What is the northernmost inhabited settlement in the UK?
   a. Skaw, Unst
   b. John O'Groats, Caithness
   c. Stromness, Mainland, Orkney

7. In which English county can you find the Royal
   Military Academy Sandhurst?
   a. Berkshire
   b. Buckinghamshire
   c. Hampshire

8. In which UK county could you find the village of Coton
   in the Elms – known for being the furthest settlement
   from a UK coast?
   a. Warwickshire
   b. Derbyshire
   c. Shropshire

9. On what river would you find the High Force waterfall?
   a. Ouse
   b. Aire
   c. Tees

10. How many countries make up the United Kingdom?
    a. 3
    b. 4
    c. 5

# CHAPTER 5

# CASE STUDY — GOING DEEPER

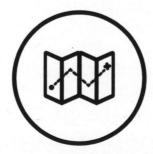

# MILITARY PLANNING

'A good plan, violently executed now, is better than a perfect plan next week.'

General George S. Patton

Individuals and groups are tasked with making decisions every day. These can vary from very simple, almost unconscious, decisions to extremely complex ones, like military operations. However, common throughout this spectrum is the generic process people go through to make a decision.

This decision-making process is the subject of a vast amount of academic and commercial literature, but at its simplest it can be reduced to four key steps:

- Define the problem
- Gather and consider information
- Identify possible solutions
- Select the best solution

This universally accepted basic problem-solving model therefore establishes the base logic for both NATO's and the British Army's formalised planning process, known as an *estimate*. However, it remains a useful reference framework for decision making in both military or civilian life.

Against the backdrop of this generic decision-making process, military estimates have been developed as a formal process to develop and make a decision on a course of action. Importantly, they are planning tools that enable military commanders to make timely and appropriate decisions, and to generate plans and orders.

The formal definition from the Allied Joint Doctrine for Operational Level Planning, 2013 is: 'The estimate is a logical process of reasoning by which the commander, faced with an ill-structured problem, arrives at a decision for a course of action to be taken in order to achieve their mission.'

The unique context of military decision making is also worthy of note at this point in that, unlike most commercial decisions, poor decisions or inefficient process in the military have the potential for the loss of life; therefore, it is vital that planning is conducted as effectively as possible. A key part is conducting planning under time pressure, with physical and mental stress and with a less than perfect knowledge of the situation.

The main estimate process used by the British Army is called the Combat Estimate (CE).

It is designed to generate plans for tactical problems that typically need urgent resolution. It assumes that the commander and planning staff of the unit or formation have a good base understanding of the situation they face and that there is no need (and no time) to analyse the broader issues. The Combat Estimate is therefore intended to make it easy to focus on what you are being called upon to do, and what decisions you need to make, all at a time when you may be under considerable stress.

The CE is divided into three stages, with simple questions to focus your analysis:

### Stage 1 – Analysis of the environment and mission:
- What is the current situation?
- What have I been told to do and why?
- What effects do I need to achieve and what direction must I give?

### Stage 2 – Development of the plan:
- Where can I best accomplish each action/effect?

- What resources do I need to accomplish each action/effect?
- Where and when do the actions/effects take place in relation to each other?
- What control measures do I need to impose?

**Stage 3 – Communication of the plan:**
- Refine the plan and communicate it through orders

It should, however, be noted that, as with all military matters, it is essential to stay flexible and adaptable. While the CE provides a planning framework, it should be adapted to meet the prevailing context.

# ARMY OFFICER SELECTION BOARD (AOSB) PRACTICE PLANNING EXERCISE

The following exercise is based on the kind of assessment that a would-be army officer might undertake during the recruitment process to test planning and decision-making abilities. Problem solving under pressure is a key skill, so this puzzle has been designed for you to solve it under timed conditions. It is shorter and simpler than the official assessment, and you should aim to complete it in about 40 minutes.

If you prefer more space than given in this book for your notes, use a large sheet of blank paper when you get to the area for your answers and planning – at an actual assessment centre you would be given a sheet of A3 paper.

When you start the task, you'll be given a briefing with some background information and then the current situation that you need to plan for. Next, you will be given some instructions, and space to write your plan.

Finally, there are some suggested plans – but don't look at these until the 40 minutes is up! You can use them to review the decisions you made yourself, and to look at some sensible solutions that have been prepared for you.

## 1. DESERT DILEMMA

### Background information

The bitter civil war in Surah (a Middle Eastern republic) continues to rumble on, leaving a trail of devastation in its wake. The general population have been left starving and prone to disease, while towns and cities in large parts of the country have ceased to function.

You have recently accepted a job as an aid coordinator (effectively the in-country second-in-command) for an internationally recognised charity, Feed, Clothe and Treat the Children (FCTC), which is currently involved in delivering both food and medical aid to all regions within Surah, especially hospitals, refugee centres and orphanages.

You arrived in the neighbouring country of Nordil (a stable constitutional monarchy with a respected and modernising king) via Queen Ellana International Airport (QEIA) a week ago. It is in Nordil that FCTC has its main depots and regional headquarters.

On arrival, you received extensive briefs and information on the situation in Surah. In essence, the civil war has been raging for several years. There are three main factions, all mutually hostile, although none is quite strong enough to decisively beat the other two:

- The Government Forces (GF) retain control of about 60 per cent of the country. They remain a generally disciplined and potent force, although international sanctions are certainly now hampering their military efficiency. The GF remain unswervingly loyal to the Al Dosti family, who have supplied Surah's leaders for the last six decades
- The GF are opposed by the Democratic Coalition (DC), a loose and generally disorganised grouping of progressive liberals seeking a Western-style democracy. In total, the DC controls around 25 per cent of the country, mostly in the far north
- The third grouping is known as the Brotherhood for the Liberation of Surah (BLS). They are an intolerant, reactionary and highly dangerous grouping of

fundamentalist extremists, who currently control around 15 per cent of the country, mostly in the north-west but also including the southern town of Courtra. They actively target Westerners for capture and have recently begun to execute those that have fallen into their hands. Travel through BLS-controlled areas should always be avoided

## Current situation

On Monday 17 July you attend a briefing at FCTC HQ in Nordil's capital Avar. You discover that the next day you will set off in a small convoy heading into Surah. The convoy will be made up of three vehicles:

- A Land Rover being driven by your boss, Sean Lang, accompanied by another co-worker, Dave Bennet
- A second Land Rover, driven by you. You will be accompanied by Clara Nazarine, the team medic (who will subsequently stay to work at the hospital in Marzil)
- The third and final vehicle will be a specialist refrigerated truck for the carriage of medicines driven by a local contractor, Abdulrahman Al Ghanim, accompanied by another team member, Jonny Jarvis

Sean explains that the convoy will head out at 0900 hrs tomorrow:

- On the good roads of Nordil, the 120 miles to the border will take three hours, but border formalities will always take an additional four hours each way, so the team will stay overnight at the refugee camp of Al Safwani on the Nordil side of the border. This camp contains a good hospital

- Next, the convoy will drive the short distance to the border, completing the crossing by 1200 hrs
- The convoy will then proceed to the strategically important town of Ramla in order to renew the FCTC licence to operate in GF-controlled areas. This must be completed by 1600 hrs on 19 July (when the GF offices shut) or the entire FCTC organisation in Surah will be forced to close. This will still allow time for the convoy to continue on the Faisal Road before joining Route 2 to the refugee centre at Marzil, where the medicines and plasma contained in the refrigerated truck must be delivered by 2000 hrs at the latest

Sean tells you that driving should be avoided after last light (currently 2130 hrs). He also warns the group that sandstorms are common at this time of year. They are likely to last for more than 24 hours. They ruin any mobile phone signal, and double travel times on all roads, while making travel on desert tracks impossible.

The next day, the convoy sets out and all starts according to plan. Having successfully crossed the border, the convoy is at 2 Mosque Junction (2MJ) when a lorry completely fails to stop at the junction and ploughs into Sean's vehicle, causing it to over-turn. The truck driver is uninjured, but both Sean and Dave are seriously injured. Dave has a broken leg but is conscious. Sean has a bad head injury, which in Clara's opinion must be treated by a neurology specialist, likely to be found only in a major hospital. She can think of just three such hospitals in the area, at Al Safwani, Khar Zubaya or Marzil. She says she can't be certain, but without proper treatment within a couple of hours Sean is likely to die.

By Sean's side is his map with some notes written on it. As you look at it, you glance up to see a sandstorm rolling in towards you. You look at your watch. It is 1230 hrs.

## Requirement
It is up to you to decide what to do next.

Using the sketch map to help you assess the problem:

1. decide your *aims*
2. and the *factors* that will affect your decisions
3. consider the *courses of action* open to you, and
4. arrive at your *plan*, giving your reasons

Note that by AOSB convention, only *movement* timings need to be considered when constructing your plan. Other actions can be considered to take zero time; so, for instance, actually dropping a casualty at a hospital takes zero time, but getting a casualty to hospital does take time.

## Aims
- Think about what *must* be achieved and by what time
- Try and order your aims in terms of priority. You might want to split them into *essential* aims and *desirable* aims to do this
- It might also be helpful to create a short 'codename' for each aim to help you when planning later on, so you can refer to things compactly and clearly – for example, your highest-priority essential aim might be referred to as E1, followed by E2, etc.

## Factors and deductions
- Look at all the information you have been given and assess what effect each issue will have on your courses

of action. For example, you could consider how information you have about weather will affect your plans
- You might want to think about time constraints, route options and what resources are available to you
- Try and summarise only what is relevant to the decisions you have to make *now* – only what is most helpful to you when planning your courses of action

### Decide courses of action

Can you come up with a course of action that achieves all of your aims, within the time constraints, and takes all of your risk factors into account? Can you create a timeline of the steps you need to take in chronological order?

- Try to come up with at least three potential courses of action. If any will not work, eliminate them as you go
- If you have mapped out the most sensible courses of action and have multiple options that you haven't already eliminated, assess them and order them in order of effectiveness

At the end of the exercise, you should choose *one* of your courses of action that you believe achieves the greatest number of aims in the time you have. This is your *plan*.

## Map

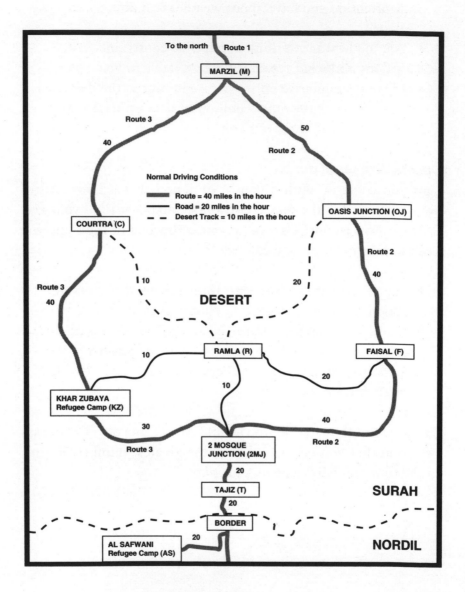

## 2. Answer Sheet

Complete the pages that follow, using the guidance on pages 204–5.

# WRITTEN PLANNING EXERCISE

### Aims:

........................................................................................................

........................................................................................................

........................................................................................................

........................................................................................................

........................................................................................................

........................................................................................................

........................................................................................................

........................................................................................................

........................................................................................................

........................................................................................................

........................................................................................................

........................................................................................................

........................................................................................................

........................................................................................................

........................................................................................................

........................................................................................................

## Factors which affect the plan/Deductions:

..................................................................................

..................................................................................

..................................................................................

..................................................................................

..................................................................................

..................................................................................

..................................................................................

..................................................................................

..................................................................................

..................................................................................

..................................................................................

..................................................................................

..................................................................................

..................................................................................

..................................................................................

..................................................................................

..................................................................................

..................................................................................

..................................................................................

**Courses of action (three should be identified), and reasons for rejecting/accepting each course of action:**

........................................................................................

........................................................................................

........................................................................................

........................................................................................

........................................................................................

........................................................................................

........................................................................................

........................................................................................

........................................................................................

........................................................................................

........................................................................................

........................................................................................

........................................................................................

........................................................................................

........................................................................................

........................................................................................

........................................................................................

........................................................................................

........................................................................................

**Plan that you adopted (including detailed timings):**

..................................................................................................

..................................................................................................

..................................................................................................

..................................................................................................

..................................................................................................

..................................................................................................

..................................................................................................

..................................................................................................

..................................................................................................

..................................................................................................

..................................................................................................

..................................................................................................

..................................................................................................

..................................................................................................

..................................................................................................

..................................................................................................

..................................................................................................

..................................................................................................

..................................................................................................

..................................................................................................

# 2. DESERT DILEMMA - POSSIBLE SOLUTION

## Aims

You should have identified all of the aims, and possibly split them into *essential* and *desirable* aims. You are unlikely to achieve all of the aims – but you should aim to at least identify the essential ones.

In priority order, and with codenames, the *essential* aims could be:

1. Stabilise casualties. **E1**
2. Get both casualties to appropriate medical facilities (Sean within two hours) therefore by 1430 hrs 19 July. **E2**
3. Renew FCTC licence in RAMLA (R) by 1600 hrs 19 July. **E3** (If FCTC is closed down, a significant number of lives will be affected)
4. Get medicines and plasma to Marzil (M) by 2000 hrs 19 July. **E4**

*Desirable* aims in priority order would be:

1. Inform FCTC of accident as soon as possible. **D1**
2. Inform GF authorities of accident as soon as possible. **D2**
3. Get Clara Nazarine to Marzil Hospital by last light. **D3**

## Factors/deductions

1. Time now 1230 hrs 19 July (journey started on 18 July, overnighted at Al Safwani – therefore it is now the 19th). Sean must be with a specialist by 1430 hrs
2. Sandstorm is just starting – likely to last for 24 hours. Speed on all routes/roads halved – desert tracks now unusable. Additionally, mobile phone comms will be unworkable. Will have to seek other comms methods

3. Last light is at 2130 hrs – has this timing become irrelevant due to sandstorm?
4. BLS in possession of Coutra (C). Travel through BLS territory should be avoided
5. Sean requires neurological care – Clara believes this will only be available at one of three locations; Al Safwani (AS), Khar Zubaya (KZ) or Marzil (M). AS is over the border – it will take at least four hours to clear the border, by which time Sean is likely to die
6. I have two vehicles – the LR and the refrigerated truck. There is nothing in my orders saying that I cannot split the convoy and undertake concurrent activity
7. *Assumption*: that comms (other than mobile phones) will be available in towns/refugee camps

## Possible courses of action

The possible courses of action below have been presented as a timeline, with abbreviations for aims and locations. Refer back to the text to clarify the various codenames and abbreviations.

### COA 1 (convoy stays together)

| Time | 1230 | 1hr | 1330 | 1hr | 1430 | 2hrs | 1630 | 2hrs | 1830 |
|------|------|-----|------|-----|------|------|------|------|------|
| Location | 2MJ | --------- | R | ------------ | KZ | ----------- | C | --------------- | M |
| Aims | E1 | | E3 | | E2 | | | | E4 |
| | | | D2/D1 | | | | | | D3 |

### COA 2 (convoy stays together)

| Time | 1230 | 1hr | 1330 | 1hr | 1430 | 1hr | 1530 | 2hrs | 1730 | 4.5hrs | 2200 |
|------|------|-----|------|-----|------|-----|------|------|------|--------|------|
| Location | 2MJ | --------- | R | ------------ | KZ | ----------- | R | -------------- | F | ----------------- | M |
| Aims | E1 | | E3 | | E2 | | | | | | E4 |
| | | | D2/D1 | | | | | | | | D3 |

E4 out of time – Reject.

## COA 3 (convoy stays together)

| Time | 1230 | 1.5hrs | 1400 | 1hr | 1500 | 2hrs | 1700 | 4.5hrs | 2130 |
|---|---|---|---|---|---|---|---|---|---|
| Location | 2MJ | -------------- | KZ----------- | | R------------ | | F---------------- | | M |
| Aims | E1 | | E2 | | E3 | | | | E4 |
| | | | D2/D1 | | | | | | D3 |

E4 out of time – Reject.

## COA 4 (convoy splits at 2MJ)

LR

| Time | 1230 | 1.5hrs | 1400 | 1hr | 1500 | 2hrs | 1700 | 4.5hrs | 2130 |
|---|---|---|---|---|---|---|---|---|---|
| Location | 2MJ | -------------- | KZ----------- | | R------------ | | F---------------- | | M |
| Aims | E1 | | E2 | | E3 | | | | D3 |
| | | | D2/D1 | | | | | | |

Truck

| Time | 1230 | 2hrs | 1430 | 4.5hrs | 1900 |
|---|---|---|---|---|---|
| Location | 2MJ | --------------- | F---------------- | | M |
| Aims | | | | E4 | |

## COA 5 (convoy splits at KZ)

LR

| Time | 1230 | 1.5hrs | 1400 | 1hr | 1500 | 1hr | 1600 | 2hrs | 1800 | 2hrs | 2000 |
|---|---|---|---|---|---|---|---|---|---|---|---|
| Location | 2MJ | -------------- | KZ----------- | | R------------ | | KZ-------------- | | C------------- | | M |
| Aims | E1 | | E2 | | E3 | | | | | | D3 |
| | | | D2/D1 | | | | | | | | |

Truck

| Time | 1230 | 1.5hrs | 1400 | 2hrs | 1600 | 2hrs | 1800 |
|---|---|---|---|---|---|---|---|
| Location | 2MJ | --------------- | KZ----------- | | C ------------ | | M |
| Aims | | | | | E4 | | |

## COA 6 (convoy splits 2MJ)

LR

| Time | 1230 | 1hr | 1330 | 1hr | 1430 | 5hrs | 1930 |
|---|---|---|---|---|---|---|---|
| Location | 2MJ | --------- | T | --------- | Border | ---------- | AS |
| Aims | E1 | | D2/D1 | | | | E2 |

Truck

| Time | 1230 | 2hrs | 1430 | 4.5hrs | 1900 |
|---|---|---|---|---|---|
| Location | 2MJ | -------------- | F | ----------------- | M |
| Aims | | | | | E4 |

E2 out of time – Sean dead. E3 not achieved. D3 not achieved – Reject.

There are various other courses – but they are all variations on one of the courses above.

### Selection of plan

Of the courses not already rejected, we are left with three courses of action that meet all of the aims in the required time-frames. These are COAs 1, 4 and 5.

## COA 1

Advantages: convoy stays together. All aims achieved by 1830 hrs.

Disadvantages: Sean not treated till 1430 hrs – cutting it very fine. Convoy routes via C – BLS controlled.

## COA 4

Advantages: Sean treated by 1400 hrs. All other aims achieved in time. Least risky option.

Disadvantages: LR only arrives at M as last light falls (2130 hrs).

**COA 5**

Advantages: Sean treated by 1400 hrs. All aims achieved by
2000 hrs.

Disadvantages: Convoy routes via C – BLS controlled.

We therefore select COA 4, since it achieves all required aims on
time and is also the least risky option, as no vehicles are routed
via C – therefore we do not run the risk of having personnel
taken hostage.

**Course that you adopted (including detailed timings)**

- Time now 1230 hrs 19 Jul. Clara and I stabilise
  casualties. Casualties then loaded onto Land Rover
  (LR). Truck with medicines and Abdulrahman and
  Jonny proceeds to Faisal on Route 2 (1430), then on to
  M, arriving at 1900 hrs
- LR with Clara and myself takes casualties to KZ. Arrive
  1400 hrs, casualties admitted to hospital. I also inform
  FCTC and GF authorities
- LR moves to R. Arrive 1500 hrs. Renew FCTC licence.
- LR continues to F and then M. Arrive 2130 hrs. All
  aims achieved

# [SOLUTIONS]

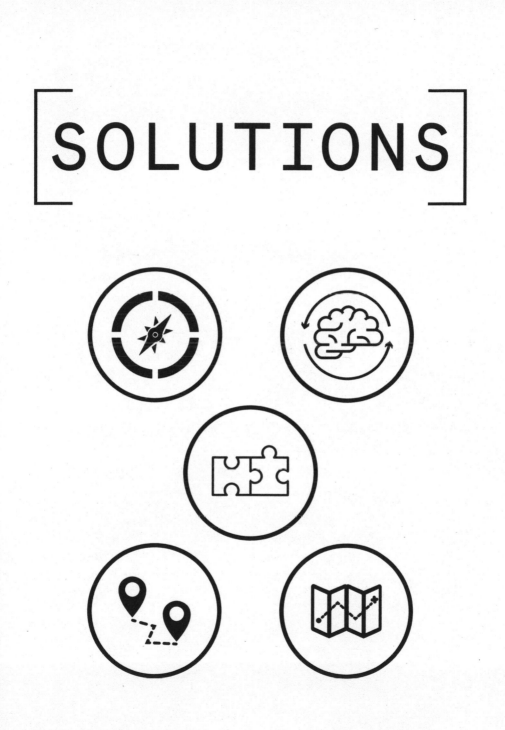

# CHAPTER 1: IN THE FIELD

## LOGICAL REASONING

### 1. Anti-poaching

- **Blue:** Jess and Michael; **animal:** Elephants
- **Green:** Elijah and Priti; **animal:** Rhinoceroses
- **Red:** Liam and Rita; **animal:** Leopards

### 2. Feeding the troops

- Monday: Chicken tikka and water
- Tuesday: Lasagne and coffee
- Wednesday: Irish stew and tea

### 3. Army protected patrol vehicles

The best vehicle is the Foxhound:

| Vehicle | Speed (mph) | Crew |
| --- | --- | --- |
| Ridgback | 56 | 3 |
| Panther | 50 | 4 |
| Foxhound | 70 | 6 |

### 4. A natural disaster

- 21 Engineer Regiment (your regiment) arrived first, followed by 17 Port and Maritime Regiment. 2 Medical Regiment arrived last
- 21 Engineer Regiment brought blankets and tents
- 17 Port and Maritime Regiment brought water sanitation kits
- 2 Medical Regiment brought temporary fencing and tools

### 5. International work

- Each service period is five months
- Jinny and Raj are both in the Falkland Islands
- Harry is in Belize

## PRACTICAL PUZZLES

### 1. Losing the light

At 1800 on 15 December in the UK, the sun would have been set for two hours, from around 4pm. There would be no shadows or daylight.

### 2. Emergency navigation

As it is 22 March, the sun will rise due east and so, at 0900, halfway between dawn and midday, the sun will be in the north-east and will cast the soldier's shadow in the opposite direction: south-west. This means that the soldier is facing north and therefore needs to about-turn 180 degrees in order to head due south and reach safety.

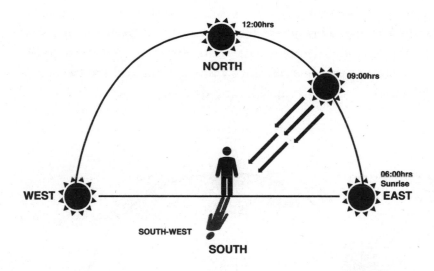

### 3. Sensible shade

The sun will rise from the east, so the location marked C will be in shade.

### 4. Sticks and stones

A line stretching east to west can be created by marking the trajectory of shadows cast by the same object over a period of time. So, if you place the stick into the sand so that it stands vertically, you can mark the top of the shadow it creates with one of the stones. Wait for at least a quarter of an hour, then mark the position of the new location of the shadow created by the stick.

Because of the sun's movement from east to west, and the shadow's movement from west to east, you know that the first stone is in the more westerly position, and the second stone the more easterly. This means that a line drawn from the first stone to the second will point east – the direction you must follow. You can use this line, once it's been drawn, and the two points East and West, to navigate in any direction.

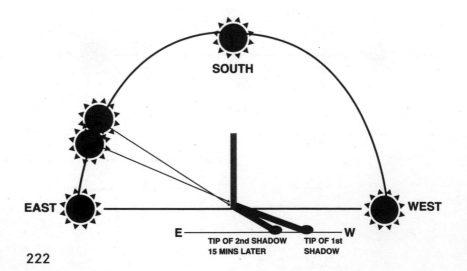

SOUTH

EAST

WEST

E

W

TIP OF 2nd SHADOW
15 MINS LATER

TIP OF 1st
SHADOW

## 5. Search area

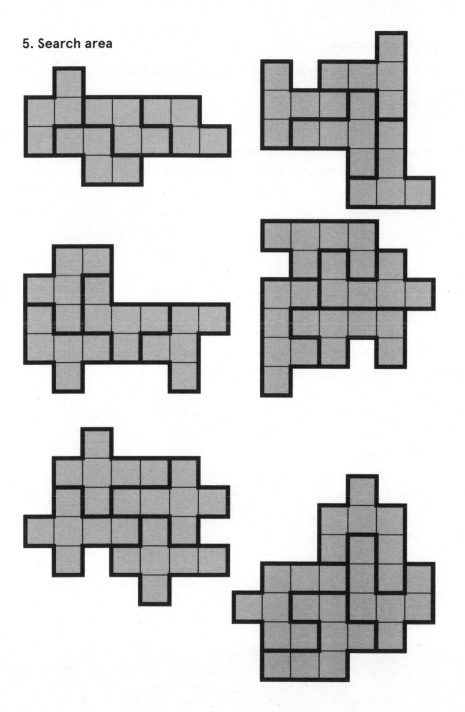

## 6. Shadow match

The correct shadow is E.

## 7. On reflection

The text reads 'MEDECINS SANS FRONTIERES' – the vehicle belongs to the medical humanitarian organisation that, in English, translates as 'Doctors Without Borders'.

# CAMOUFLAGE AND NIGHT VISION

## 1. Rapid differences

## 2. Subtler differences

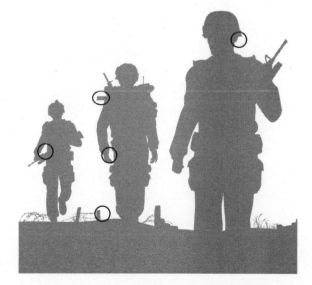

## 3. Night navigation

# MAZES AND NAVIGATION

### 1. Star maze

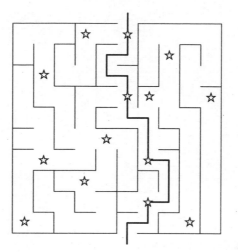

Four stars.

### 2. Left-turn maze

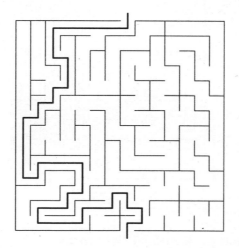

Fourteen left turns.

### 3. Stars and diamonds maze

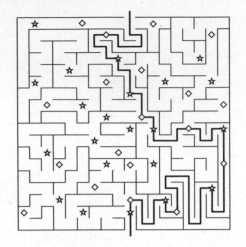

Seven stars and six diamonds.

### 4. Left- and right-turn maze

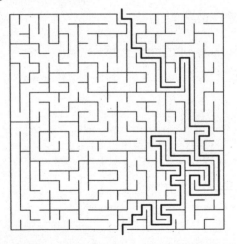

Twenty-four left turns and 24 right turns.

Since the entrance is directly above the exit, and turns are always 90 degrees, the number of left and right turns must be equal; otherwise you would not end up pointing in the correct direction. Put another way, every right turn must cancel out a left turn, and vice versa. This is true only because there are no loops in this maze, or any way of crossing over or under the path.

## 5. Under-bridge maze

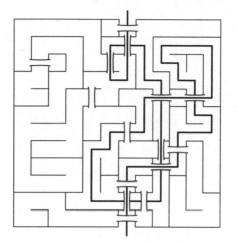

The path goes under 11 bridges.

## 6. Over-bridge maze

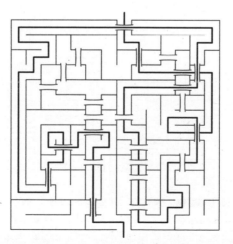

The path crosses over 10 bridges.

### 7. Under- and over-bridge maze

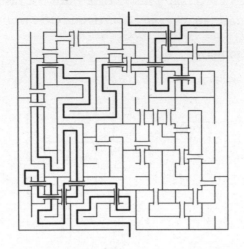

The path goes under and over a total of 14 different bridges.

### 8. Under- or over-bridge maze

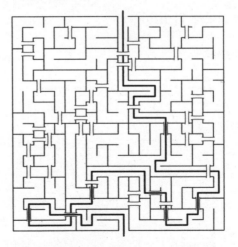

The path goes under seven bridges and crosses over seven bridges.

### 9. Find your supplies

A is your starting point; D is your drop-off point.

### 10. Setting up camp

The most suitable campsite is B, which is on level ground, close to a road, river and footpath, and located on a valley floor, giving it natural shelter. Other options are less good, since A is close to several permanent settlements; C, while close to water and transport links, is located on the side of a steep hill; and D is located on top of a hill and therefore exposed to elements.

## 11. Tents

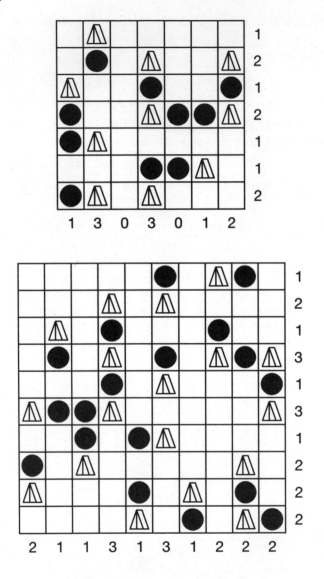

## 12. Grid references – standard

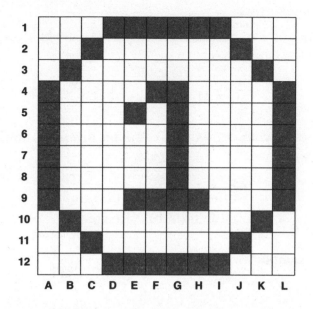

Congratulations! You've uncovered a first-place medal.

## 13. Grid references – four-digit

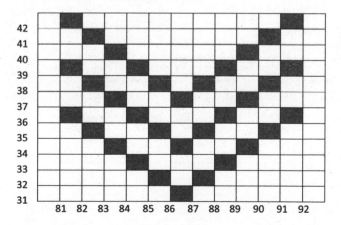

You have drawn three chevrons, which indicate the rank of *sergeant* in the British Army.

## MAP SCALES

### 1. Photo intelligence

To calculate scale, according to the GSM triangle, you use the equation $S = G \div M$, so:

$$G \div M = 100 \text{ m} \div 16 \text{ mm}.$$

First, convert your values to a common denomination, such as centimetres:

$$100 \text{ m x } 100 = 10,000 \text{ cm}$$
$$16 \text{ mm} \div 10 = 1.6 \text{ cm}.$$

So your equation is:

$$S = 10,000 \div 1.6$$
$$S = 6,250.$$

$$\text{Scale} = 1{:}6,250.$$

### 2. Scale calculations

| | Map Distance | Ground Distance | Scale |
|---|---|---|---|
| a) | 20 cm | 60 km | 1:300,000 |
| b) | 50 mm | 250 m | 1:5,000 |
| c) | 4 cm | 8 km | 1:200,000 |
| d) | 14 mm | 5,600 m | 1:400,000 |
| e) | 2.8 cm | 140 m | 1:5,000 |

## 3. Ground-distance calculations

| | Map Distance | Scale | Ground Distance |
|---|---|---|---|
| a) | 3.7 cm | 1:25,000 | 925 m |
| b) | 45 mm | 1:100,000 | 4.5 km |
| c) | 8 cm | 1:40,000 | 3.2 km |
| d) | 2.4 cm | 1:12,000 | 288 m |
| e) | 38 mm | 1:250,000 | 9.5 km |

## 4. Map-distance calculations

| | Ground Distance | Scale | Map Distance |
|---|---|---|---|
| a) | 2.8 km | 1:5,000 | 56 cm |
| b) | 450 m | 1:50,000 | 9 mm |
| c) | 7.5 km | 1:20,000 | 37.5 cm |
| d) | 700 m | 1:2,500 | 28 cm |
| e) | 32 km | 1:250,000 | 12.8 cm |

# CHAPTER 2: COGNITIVE TESTING

## SUDOKU

### 1. Sudoku 9x9

| 1 | 9 | 7 | 4 | 8 | 2 | 5 | 6 | 3 |
|---|---|---|---|---|---|---|---|---|
| 5 | 8 | 2 | 3 | 7 | 6 | 4 | 1 | 9 |
| 3 | 6 | 4 | 9 | 1 | 5 | 7 | 2 | 8 |
| 8 | 7 | 6 | 1 | 5 | 4 | 3 | 9 | 2 |
| 4 | 1 | 3 | 8 | 2 | 9 | 6 | 7 | 5 |
| 9 | 2 | 5 | 6 | 3 | 7 | 1 | 8 | 4 |
| 6 | 3 | 9 | 7 | 4 | 8 | 2 | 5 | 1 |
| 7 | 5 | 1 | 2 | 9 | 3 | 8 | 4 | 6 |
| 2 | 4 | 8 | 5 | 6 | 1 | 9 | 3 | 7 |

### 2. Sudoku 6x6

| 5 | 6 | 1 | 2 | 4 | 3 |
|---|---|---|---|---|---|
| 4 | 3 | 2 | 6 | 1 | 5 |
| 3 | 4 | 5 | 1 | 6 | 2 |
| 2 | 1 | 6 | 5 | 3 | 4 |
| 1 | 2 | 4 | 3 | 5 | 6 |
| 6 | 5 | 3 | 4 | 2 | 1 |

### 3. Latin square

| 2 | 4 | 1 | 3 | 6 | 5 |
|---|---|---|---|---|---|
| 4 | 2 | 6 | 5 | 3 | 1 |
| 1 | 3 | 5 | 2 | 4 | 6 |
| 5 | 6 | 3 | 4 | 1 | 2 |
| 3 | 1 | 2 | 6 | 5 | 4 |
| 6 | 5 | 4 | 1 | 2 | 3 |

## 4. Touchy

| 4 | 6 | 1 | 2 | 5 | 3 |
|---|---|---|---|---|---|
| 1 | 5 | 3 | 4 | 6 | 2 |
| 3 | 2 | 6 | 5 | 1 | 4 |
| 6 | 1 | 4 | 3 | 2 | 5 |
| 2 | 3 | 5 | 1 | 4 | 6 |
| 5 | 4 | 2 | 6 | 3 | 1 |

## 5. Touch sudoku

| 3 | 6 | 4 | 1 | 5 | 2 |
|---|---|---|---|---|---|
| 2 | 1 | 5 | 6 | 4 | 3 |
| 5 | 4 | 2 | 3 | 1 | 6 |
| 1 | 3 | 6 | 4 | 2 | 5 |
| 6 | 2 | 1 | 5 | 3 | 4 |
| 4 | 5 | 3 | 2 | 6 | 1 |

## 6. Two-step diagonal sudoku

| 3 | 4 | 6 | 2 | 5 | 1 |
|---|---|---|---|---|---|
| 1 | 2 | 5 | 4 | 3 | 6 |
| 5 | 3 | 1 | 6 | 2 | 4 |
| 4 | 6 | 2 | 3 | 1 | 5 |
| 2 | 1 | 4 | 5 | 6 | 3 |
| 6 | 5 | 3 | 1 | 4 | 2 |

## 7. Diagonal sudoku

| 1 | 4 | 6 | 5 | 3 | 2 |
|---|---|---|---|---|---|
| 2 | 3 | 5 | 6 | 4 | 1 |
| 4 | 5 | 2 | 1 | 6 | 3 |
| 6 | 1 | 3 | 4 | 2 | 5 |
| 3 | 6 | 1 | 2 | 5 | 4 |
| 5 | 2 | 4 | 3 | 1 | 6 |

## 8. Regional sudoku

| 1 | 6 | 5 | 4 | 2 | 3 |
|---|---|---|---|---|---|
| 4 | 3 | 2 | 6 | 1 | 5 |
| 6 | 1 | 4 | 5 | 3 | 2 |
| 5 | 2 | 3 | 1 | 6 | 4 |
| 3 | 4 | 1 | 2 | 5 | 6 |
| 2 | 5 | 6 | 3 | 4 | 1 |

## 9. Jigsaw sudoku

| 2 | 5 | 6 | 3 | 4 | 1 |
|---|---|---|---|---|---|
| 3 | 4 | 1 | 5 | 6 | 2 |
| 6 | 3 | 4 | 2 | 1 | 5 |
| 1 | 2 | 3 | 6 | 5 | 4 |
| 5 | 1 | 2 | 4 | 3 | 6 |
| 4 | 6 | 5 | 1 | 2 | 3 |

## 10. Wrap-around sudoku

| 2 | 5 | 4 | 6 | 1 | 3 |
|---|---|---|---|---|---|
| 3 | 6 | 1 | 2 | 4 | 5 |
| 6 | 2 | 5 | 4 | 3 | 1 |
| 4 | 1 | 3 | 5 | 2 | 6 |
| 5 | 3 | 2 | 1 | 6 | 4 |
| 1 | 4 | 6 | 3 | 5 | 2 |

## 11. Wrap-around boxed sudoku

| 6 | 2 | 3 | 5 | 4 | 1 |
|---|---|---|---|---|---|
| 5 | 4 | 1 | 6 | 3 | 2 |
| 2 | 3 | 6 | 1 | 5 | 4 |
| 1 | 5 | 4 | 2 | 6 | 3 |
| 3 | 6 | 2 | 4 | 1 | 5 |
| 4 | 1 | 5 | 3 | 2 | 6 |

## REVENGE OF SUDOKU

### 1. Sudoku

| 3 | 8 | 5 | 4 | 6 | 7 | 2 | 9 | 1 |
| 1 | 4 | 9 | 2 | 8 | 5 | 7 | 6 | 3 |
| 6 | 2 | 7 | 3 | 9 | 1 | 4 | 5 | 8 |
| 8 | 7 | 6 | 9 | 2 | 3 | 5 | 1 | 4 |
| 2 | 9 | 3 | 1 | 5 | 4 | 6 | 8 | 7 |
| 4 | 5 | 1 | 6 | 7 | 8 | 9 | 3 | 2 |
| 7 | 1 | 2 | 5 | 3 | 6 | 8 | 4 | 9 |
| 5 | 3 | 8 | 7 | 4 | 9 | 1 | 2 | 6 |
| 9 | 6 | 4 | 8 | 1 | 2 | 3 | 7 | 5 |

### 2. Outside sudoku

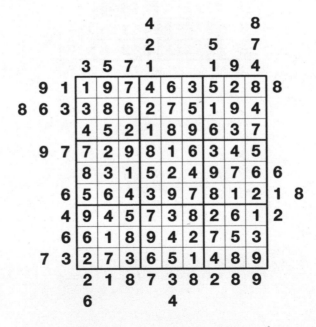

## 3. Quad clue sudoku

| 5 | 3 | 7 | 8 | 6 | 1 | 9 | 2 | 4 |
|---|---|---|---|---|---|---|---|---|
| 9 | 6 | 1 | 2 | 7 | 4 | 8 | 5 | 3 |
| 4 | 8 | 2 | 3 | 9 | 5 | 1 | 7 | 6 |
| 2 | 9 | 3 | 7 | 8 | 6 | 4 | 1 | 5 |
| 1 | 4 | 8 | 5 | 3 | 2 | 7 | 6 | 9 |
| 6 | 7 | 5 | 1 | 4 | 9 | 3 | 8 | 2 |
| 7 | 5 | 4 | 6 | 1 | 3 | 2 | 9 | 8 |
| 3 | 1 | 6 | 9 | 2 | 8 | 5 | 4 | 7 |
| 8 | 2 | 9 | 4 | 5 | 7 | 6 | 3 | 1 |

## 4. Trio sudoku

| 5 | 3 | 4 | 7 | 8 | 1 | 6 | 9 | 2 |
|---|---|---|---|---|---|---|---|---|
| 7 | 8 | 1 | 2 | 9 | 6 | 3 | 5 | 4 |
| 6 | 2 | 9 | 4 | 5 | 3 | 7 | 1 | 8 |
| 3 | 1 | 2 | 8 | 4 | 7 | 9 | 6 | 5 |
| 9 | 6 | 7 | 3 | 2 | 5 | 4 | 8 | 1 |
| 4 | 5 | 8 | 6 | 1 | 9 | 2 | 3 | 7 |
| 8 | 7 | 6 | 1 | 3 | 2 | 5 | 4 | 9 |
| 2 | 4 | 5 | 9 | 6 | 8 | 1 | 7 | 3 |
| 1 | 9 | 3 | 5 | 7 | 4 | 8 | 2 | 6 |

## 5. Frame sudoku

|     | 17 | 11 | 17 | 24 | 12 | 9 | 15 | 11 | 19 |     |
|-----|----|----|----|----|----|---|----|----|----|-----|
| 8   | 1  | 3  | 4  | 8  | 2  | 5 | 6  | 7  | 9  | 22  |
| 21  | 7  | 6  | 8  | 9  | 4  | 3 | 5  | 1  | 2  | 8   |
| 16  | 9  | 2  | 5  | 7  | 6  | 1 | 4  | 3  | 8  | 15  |
| 24  | 8  | 9  | 7  | 6  | 3  | 2 | 1  | 5  | 4  | 10  |
| 7   | 4  | 1  | 2  | 5  | 7  | 9 | 3  | 8  | 6  | 17  |
| 14  | 6  | 5  | 3  | 1  | 8  | 4 | 2  | 9  | 7  | 18  |
| 20  | 3  | 8  | 9  | 4  | 5  | 6 | 7  | 2  | 1  | 10  |
| 18  | 5  | 7  | 6  | 2  | 1  | 8 | 9  | 4  | 3  | 16  |
| 7   | 2  | 4  | 1  | 3  | 9  | 7 | 8  | 6  | 5  | 19  |
|     | 10 | 19 | 16 | 9  | 15 | 21| 24 | 12 | 9  |     |

## 6. Arrow sudoku

| 7 | 5 | 3 | 1 | 9 | 4 | 8 | 2 | 6 |
|---|---|---|---|---|---|---|---|---|
| 1 | 6 | 4 | 2 | 7 | 8 | 3 | 9 | 5 |
| 9 | 2 | 8 | 5 | 6 | 3 | 7 | 4 | 1 |
| 5 | 8 | 7 | 4 | 3 | 9 | 6 | 1 | 2 |
| 4 | 9 | 2 | 8 | 1 | 6 | 5 | 7 | 3 |
| 6 | 3 | 1 | 7 | 5 | 2 | 4 | 8 | 9 |
| 2 | 1 | 6 | 3 | 4 | 7 | 9 | 5 | 8 |
| 3 | 7 | 5 | 9 | 8 | 1 | 2 | 6 | 4 |
| 8 | 4 | 9 | 6 | 2 | 5 | 1 | 3 | 7 |

## 7. Diagonal-sum sudoku

```
        42  31  25  17  28  20  7   6
      ┌───────────────────────────────┐
      │ 5   4   1   7   2   9   8   3   6 │ 32
    5 │ 6   2   7   8   3   1   9   5   4 │ 25
   10 │ 8   3   9   6   5   4   2   1   7 │ 43
   11 │ 2   6   8   1   7   5   3   4   9 │ 26
   19 │ 4   1   3   9   6   2   5   7   8 │ 22
   29 │ 9   7   5   4   8   3   6   2   1 │ 12
   36 │ 3   9   6   2   1   7   4   8   5 │ 11
   28 │ 1   5   4   3   9   8   7   6   2 │ 3
   47 │ 7   8   2   5   4   6   1   9   3 │
      └───────────────────────────────┘
         7   9   10  27  24  25  31  57
```

## 8. Sum sudoku

```
┌─────────┬─────────┬─────────┐
│ 1  9  6 │ 5  8  4 │ 3  7  2 │
│ 8  3  2 │ 1  7  6 │ 4  9  5 │
│ 4  7  5 │ 3  2  9 │ 6  1  8 │
├─────────┼─────────┼─────────┤
│ 6  4  3 │ 9  1  2 │ 8  5  7 │
│ 2  5  1 │ 7  6  8 │ 9  4  3 │
│ 9  8  7 │ 4  5  3 │ 1  2  6 │
├─────────┼─────────┼─────────┤
│ 3  6  4 │ 2  9  7 │ 5  8  1 │
│ 5  2  9 │ 8  3  1 │ 7  6  4 │
│ 7  1  8 │ 6  4  5 │ 2  3  9 │
└─────────┴─────────┴─────────┘
```

## 9. Killer sudoku

| 9 | 8 | 5 | 4 | 3 | 1 | 7 | 6 | 2 |
| 7 | 3 | 2 | 6 | 9 | 8 | 1 | 5 | 4 |
| 4 | 6 | 1 | 5 | 2 | 7 | 8 | 9 | 3 |
| 3 | 7 | 6 | 1 | 4 | 9 | 5 | 2 | 8 |
| 8 | 5 | 4 | 2 | 7 | 3 | 6 | 1 | 9 |
| 2 | 1 | 9 | 8 | 5 | 6 | 3 | 4 | 7 |
| 5 | 2 | 8 | 7 | 1 | 4 | 9 | 3 | 6 |
| 1 | 9 | 7 | 3 | 6 | 2 | 4 | 8 | 5 |
| 6 | 4 | 3 | 9 | 8 | 5 | 2 | 7 | 1 |

## 10. Killer pro sudoku

| 7 | 1 | 6 | 2 | 4 | 9 | 8 | 3 | 5 |
| 2 | 9 | 5 | 8 | 3 | 1 | 7 | 4 | 6 |
| 3 | 4 | 8 | 6 | 7 | 5 | 9 | 1 | 2 |
| 1 | 7 | 4 | 5 | 8 | 3 | 6 | 2 | 9 |
| 8 | 3 | 2 | 9 | 6 | 7 | 1 | 5 | 4 |
| 6 | 5 | 9 | 4 | 1 | 2 | 3 | 8 | 7 |
| 9 | 8 | 1 | 7 | 2 | 4 | 5 | 6 | 3 |
| 5 | 2 | 3 | 1 | 9 | 6 | 4 | 7 | 8 |
| 4 | 6 | 7 | 3 | 5 | 8 | 2 | 9 | 1 |

## 11. Mystery killer pro sudoku

| 7 | 6 | 4 | 9 | 8 | 2 | 5 | 1 | 3 |
|---|---|---|---|---|---|---|---|---|
| 5 | 8 | 3 | 1 | 7 | 4 | 6 | 9 | 2 |
| 1 | 2 | 9 | 6 | 5 | 3 | 7 | 8 | 4 |
| 6 | 1 | 7 | 4 | 3 | 8 | 2 | 5 | 9 |
| 2 | 9 | 8 | 5 | 1 | 7 | 4 | 3 | 6 |
| 3 | 4 | 5 | 2 | 6 | 9 | 8 | 7 | 1 |
| 9 | 5 | 6 | 8 | 2 | 1 | 3 | 4 | 7 |
| 8 | 7 | 1 | 3 | 4 | 6 | 9 | 2 | 5 |
| 4 | 3 | 2 | 7 | 9 | 5 | 1 | 6 | 8 |

## 12. Killer sudoku 0-8

| 2 | 6 | 4 | 8 | 1 | 7 | 0 | 5 | 3 |
|---|---|---|---|---|---|---|---|---|
| 3 | 8 | 0 | 4 | 2 | 5 | 7 | 6 | 1 |
| 7 | 1 | 5 | 3 | 0 | 6 | 8 | 2 | 4 |
| 1 | 0 | 6 | 5 | 3 | 2 | 4 | 7 | 8 |
| 8 | 4 | 2 | 7 | 6 | 0 | 1 | 3 | 5 |
| 5 | 3 | 7 | 1 | 8 | 4 | 2 | 0 | 6 |
| 0 | 7 | 8 | 6 | 4 | 3 | 5 | 1 | 2 |
| 4 | 5 | 3 | 2 | 7 | 1 | 6 | 8 | 0 |
| 6 | 2 | 1 | 0 | 5 | 8 | 3 | 4 | 7 |

## 13. Mystery killer pro sudoku 0–8

| | | | | | | | | |
|---|---|---|---|---|---|---|---|---|
| ⌜12?⌝4 | 3 | ⌜8?⌝8 | ⌜0?⌝1 | 0 | ⌜42?⌝7 | 2 | ⌜2?⌝5 | ⌜6?⌝6 |
| ⌜12?⌝2 | 6 | 0 | 8 | ⌜1?⌝5 | 4 | 3 | 7 | 1 |
| ⌜1?⌝5 | ⌜8?⌝7 | 1 | ⌜2?⌝3 | ⌜8?⌝2 | 6 | ⌜32?⌝8 | 4 | ⌜2?⌝0 |
| 1 | ⌜1?⌝4 | 3 | 5 | ⌜14?⌝6 | ⌜8?⌝0 | ⌜28?⌝7 | ⌜48?⌝8 | 2 |
| 7 | ⌜2?⌝0 | ⌜30?⌝5 | ⌜2?⌝2 | 1 | 8 | 4 | 6 | ⌜120?⌝3 |
| ⌜11?⌝8 | 2 | 6 | 4 | 7 | ⌜42?⌝3 | ⌜1?⌝0 | 1 | 5 |
| 3 | ⌜35?⌝5 | 7 | ⌜42?⌝0 | 4 | 1 | ⌜12?⌝6 | 2 | 8 |
| ⌜6?⌝0 | ⌜8?⌝1 | ⌜13?⌝4 | ⌜2?⌝6 | 8 | ⌜10?⌝2 | ⌜5?⌝5 | ⌜10?⌝3 | 7 |
| 6 | 8 | 2 | 7 | 3 | 5 | 1 | ⌜0?⌝0 | 4 |

246

# UNEQUAL SUDOKU

### 1. Futoshiki

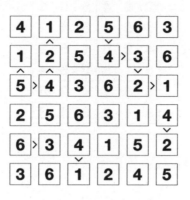

### 2. Full Futoshiki

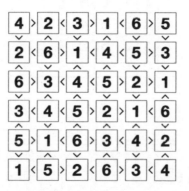

### 3. Full inequality sudoku

### 4. Inequality sudoku

| 2 | 6 | 4 | 5 | 3 | 1 |
|---|---|---|---|---|---|
| 1 | 5 | 3 | 6 | 4 | 2 |
| 4 | 2 | 6 | 1 | 5 | 3 |
| 3 | 1 | 5 | 2 | 6 | 4 |
| 6 | 3 | 1 | 4 | 2 | 5 |
| 5 | 4 | 2 | 3 | 1 | 6 |

### 5. Quad-max sudoku 6x6

| 5 | 1 | 3 | 6 | 2 | 4 |
|---|---|---|---|---|---|
| 6 | 4 | 2 | 1 | 3 | 5 |
| 4 | 2 | 1 | 5 | 6 | 3 |
| 3 | 5 | 6 | 4 | 1 | 2 |
| 1 | 3 | 5 | 2 | 4 | 6 |
| 2 | 6 | 4 | 3 | 5 | 1 |

### 6. Quad-max sudoku 9x9

| 8 | 7 | 1 | 9 | 5 | 6 | 4 | 2 | 3 |
|---|---|---|---|---|---|---|---|---|
| 9 | 2 | 4 | 1 | 3 | 8 | 7 | 5 | 6 |
| 3 | 6 | 5 | 7 | 2 | 4 | 9 | 1 | 8 |
| 6 | 4 | 7 | 5 | 8 | 2 | 1 | 3 | 9 |
| 2 | 3 | 9 | 4 | 6 | 1 | 5 | 8 | 7 |
| 1 | 5 | 8 | 3 | 7 | 9 | 2 | 6 | 4 |
| 7 | 1 | 3 | 8 | 9 | 5 | 6 | 4 | 2 |
| 5 | 9 | 2 | 6 | 4 | 3 | 8 | 7 | 1 |
| 4 | 8 | 6 | 2 | 1 | 7 | 3 | 9 | 5 |

## 7. Thermometer sudoku

| 2 | 7 | 8 | 5 | 6 | 4 | 1 | 3 | 9 |
|---|---|---|---|---|---|---|---|---|
| 5 | 9 | 6 | 7 | 3 | 1 | 2 | 8 | 4 |
| 1 | 3 | 4 | 8 | 2 | 9 | 7 | 5 | 6 |
| 7 | 2 | 9 | 4 | 1 | 8 | 3 | 6 | 5 |
| 3 | 4 | 1 | 6 | 5 | 2 | 9 | 7 | 8 |
| 8 | 6 | 5 | 3 | 9 | 7 | 4 | 1 | 2 |
| 6 | 5 | 7 | 9 | 4 | 3 | 8 | 2 | 1 |
| 4 | 8 | 2 | 1 | 7 | 6 | 5 | 9 | 3 |
| 9 | 1 | 3 | 2 | 8 | 5 | 6 | 4 | 7 |

## 8. Creasing sudoku

| 9 | 6 | 7 | 2 | 1 | 5 | 3 | 8 | 4 |
|---|---|---|---|---|---|---|---|---|
| 1 | 5 | 8 | 4 | 3 | 9 | 2 | 6 | 7 |
| 3 | 2 | 4 | 6 | 7 | 8 | 5 | 9 | 1 |
| 5 | 9 | 1 | 3 | 2 | 4 | 8 | 7 | 6 |
| 8 | 4 | 6 | 5 | 9 | 7 | 1 | 3 | 2 |
| 2 | 7 | 3 | 1 | 8 | 6 | 9 | 4 | 5 |
| 7 | 1 | 2 | 8 | 6 | 3 | 4 | 5 | 9 |
| 4 | 3 | 9 | 7 | 5 | 1 | 6 | 2 | 8 |
| 6 | 8 | 5 | 9 | 4 | 2 | 7 | 1 | 3 |

## 9. Worm sudoku

| | | | | | | | | |
|---|---|---|---|---|---|---|---|---|
| 7 | 3 | 1 | 5 | 4 | 2 | 9 | 8 | 6 |
| 8 | 6 | 4 | 1 | 7 | 9 | 5 | 2 | 3 |
| 2 | 5 | 9 | 8 | 3 | 6 | 7 | 4 | 1 |
| 5 | 4 | 6 | 9 | 1 | 8 | 3 | 7 | 2 |
| 9 | 7 | 2 | 3 | 6 | 4 | 1 | 5 | 8 |
| 3 | 1 | 8 | 7 | 2 | 5 | 4 | 6 | 9 |
| 6 | 2 | 5 | 4 | 9 | 1 | 8 | 3 | 7 |
| 1 | 8 | 3 | 6 | 5 | 7 | 2 | 9 | 4 |
| 4 | 9 | 7 | 2 | 8 | 3 | 6 | 1 | 5 |

## 10. Headless worm sudoku

| | | | | | | | | |
|---|---|---|---|---|---|---|---|---|
| 7 | 2 | 8 | 4 | 1 | 9 | 3 | 5 | 6 |
| 6 | 4 | 3 | 2 | 5 | 7 | 8 | 9 | 1 |
| 1 | 9 | 5 | 8 | 3 | 6 | 7 | 2 | 4 |
| 9 | 8 | 6 | 5 | 7 | 4 | 2 | 1 | 3 |
| 3 | 5 | 2 | 9 | 8 | 1 | 6 | 4 | 7 |
| 4 | 7 | 1 | 6 | 2 | 3 | 5 | 8 | 9 |
| 5 | 3 | 4 | 7 | 9 | 2 | 1 | 6 | 8 |
| 2 | 1 | 9 | 3 | 6 | 8 | 4 | 7 | 5 |
| 8 | 6 | 7 | 1 | 4 | 5 | 9 | 3 | 2 |

## 11. Snake sudoku

| 4 | 3 | 2 | 7 | 9 | 8 | 1 | 5 | 6 |
|---|---|---|---|---|---|---|---|---|
| 5 | 1 | 8 | 3 | 6 | 2 | 4 | 7 | 9 |
| 7 | 6 | 9 | 1 | 4 | 5 | 8 | 2 | 3 |
| 8 | 9 | 5 | 2 | 3 | 1 | 6 | 4 | 7 |
| 2 | 4 | 6 | 9 | 5 | 7 | 3 | 1 | 8 |
| 1 | 7 | 3 | 6 | 8 | 4 | 2 | 9 | 5 |
| 6 | 2 | 1 | 8 | 7 | 9 | 5 | 3 | 4 |
| 3 | 5 | 7 | 4 | 1 | 6 | 9 | 8 | 2 |
| 9 | 8 | 4 | 5 | 2 | 3 | 7 | 6 | 1 |

## 12. Consecutive sudoku

| 2 | 7 | 1 | 6 | 5 | 8 | 4 | 9 | 3 |
|---|---|---|---|---|---|---|---|---|
| 9 | 5 | 3 | 4 | 7 | 1 | 2 | 8 | 6 |
| 8 | 4 | 6 | 9 | 2 | 3 | 5 | 1 | 7 |
| 1 | 3 | 7 | 2 | 8 | 5 | 9 | 6 | 4 |
| 4 | 2 | 5 | 7 | 9 | 6 | 1 | 3 | 8 |
| 6 | 9 | 8 | 3 | 1 | 4 | 7 | 2 | 5 |
| 3 | 6 | 9 | 5 | 4 | 2 | 8 | 7 | 1 |
| 5 | 8 | 2 | 1 | 6 | 7 | 3 | 4 | 9 |
| 7 | 1 | 4 | 8 | 3 | 9 | 6 | 5 | 2 |

### 13. Kropki sudoku

| 8 | 7 | 4 | 9 | 3 | 6 | 1 | 5 | 2 |
|---|---|---|---|---|---|---|---|---|
| 9 | 2 | 1 | 4 | 5 | 7 | 3 | 8 | 6 |
| 5 | 6 | 3 | 1 | 8 | 2 | 4 | 9 | 7 |
| 7 | 9 | 8 | 6 | 1 | 3 | 2 | 4 | 5 |
| 2 | 1 | 5 | 7 | 4 | 9 | 8 | 6 | 3 |
| 4 | 3 | 6 | 5 | 2 | 8 | 7 | 1 | 9 |
| 1 | 4 | 7 | 3 | 9 | 5 | 6 | 2 | 8 |
| 6 | 5 | 2 | 8 | 7 | 1 | 9 | 3 | 4 |
| 3 | 8 | 9 | 2 | 6 | 4 | 5 | 7 | 1 |

### 14. XV sudoku

| 6 | 9 | 3 | 1 | 2 | 5 | 7 | 8 | 4 |
|---|---|---|---|---|---|---|---|---|
| 8 | 4 | 7 | 9 | 3 | 6 | 5 | 1 | 2 |
| 5 | 1 | 2 | 7 | 4 | 8 | 3 | 9 | 6 |
| 4 | 7 | 1 | 3 | 6 | 9 | 2 | 5 | 8 |
| 2 | 6 | 8 | 4 | 5 | 1 | 9 | 3 | 7 |
| 3 | 5 | 9 | 8 | 7 | 2 | 4 | 6 | 1 |
| 9 | 8 | 5 | 2 | 1 | 4 | 6 | 7 | 3 |
| 7 | 2 | 6 | 5 | 8 | 3 | 1 | 4 | 9 |
| 1 | 3 | 4 | 6 | 9 | 7 | 8 | 2 | 5 |

## 15. Anti-XV sudoku

| 1 | 8 | 6 | 3 | 9 | 7 | 4 | 2 | 5 |
|---|---|---|---|---|---|---|---|---|
| 5 | 9 | 7 | 4 | 2 | 6 | 3 | 1 | 8 |
| 3 | 4 | 2 | 5 | 1 | 8 | 9 | 7 | 6 |
| 6 | 3 | 4 | 2 | 5 | 9 | 7 | 8 | 1 |
| 9 | 5 | 8 | 1 | 7 | 4 | 2 | 6 | 3 |
| 2 | 7 | 1 | 6 | 8 | 3 | 5 | 9 | 4 |
| 7 | 1 | 3 | 9 | 6 | 5 | 8 | 4 | 2 |
| 4 | 2 | 9 | 8 | 3 | 1 | 6 | 5 | 7 |
| 8 | 6 | 5 | 7 | 4 | 2 | 1 | 3 | 9 |

## 16. Non-consecutive sudoku

| 7 | 4 | 6 | 3 | 1 | 8 | 5 | 9 | 2 |
|---|---|---|---|---|---|---|---|---|
| 2 | 8 | 3 | 5 | 9 | 4 | 7 | 1 | 6 |
| 9 | 1 | 5 | 7 | 2 | 6 | 3 | 8 | 4 |
| 1 | 5 | 9 | 4 | 6 | 2 | 8 | 3 | 7 |
| 4 | 7 | 2 | 8 | 3 | 5 | 1 | 6 | 9 |
| 6 | 3 | 8 | 1 | 7 | 9 | 4 | 2 | 5 |
| 8 | 6 | 1 | 9 | 4 | 7 | 2 | 5 | 3 |
| 5 | 2 | 4 | 6 | 8 | 3 | 9 | 7 | 1 |
| 3 | 9 | 7 | 2 | 5 | 1 | 6 | 4 | 8 |

**17. Sudoku**

| 1 | 7 | 4 | 2 | 5 | 8 | 6 | 3 | 9 |
|---|---|---|---|---|---|---|---|---|
| 8 | 2 | 9 | 6 | 4 | 3 | 1 | 7 | 5 |
| 3 | 6 | 5 | 7 | 1 | 9 | 8 | 2 | 4 |
| 6 | 3 | 8 | 1 | 9 | 5 | 2 | 4 | 7 |
| 9 | 5 | 1 | 4 | 2 | 7 | 3 | 8 | 6 |
| 2 | 4 | 7 | 3 | 8 | 6 | 9 | 5 | 1 |
| 7 | 8 | 6 | 9 | 3 | 4 | 5 | 1 | 2 |
| 4 | 1 | 3 | 5 | 6 | 2 | 7 | 9 | 8 |
| 5 | 9 | 2 | 8 | 7 | 1 | 4 | 6 | 3 |

## AND FINALLY
They were all prime numbers: 11, 13 and 17.

# CHAPTER 4: SURVIVAL

## SPEED PUZZLES
## WORD CIRCLE 1

The word that uses all the letters is **adventure**. Other words to be found include advent, advert, and, anted, ardent, averted, dare, darn, dart, date, daunt, dean, dear, deer, den, denature, dent, deter, due, duet, dun, dune, duvet, earned, end, endear, endue, endure, evade, natured, neared, need, nerved, nude, ranted, rated, raved, ravened, read, red, reed, rend, rented, rude, rued, tared, teared, teed, tend, tender, tenured, trade, tread, treed, trend, trued, tundra, tuned, turned, under, unread, urned, vaunted, vend, vented, ventured and verdant.

## WORD CIRCLE 2
The word that uses all the letters is **discovery**. Other words to be found include cider, ciders, cod, code, codes, cods, cord, cords, core, cored, cores, cosier, cosy, cove, cover, covers, coves, covey, coveys, coy, coyer, cried, cries, cry, decoy, decoys, decry, descry, dice, dices, disc, disco, discover, divorce, divorces, doc, docs, ice, iced, ices, icy, rice, riced, rices, score, scored, scrod, sic, vice, viceroy, viceroys, vices, voice, voiced and voices.

## WORD LADDER 1

ARMY ARMS AIMS AIDS BIDS BEDS

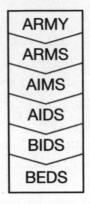

## WORD LADDER 2

CAMP CARP CARD CORD FORD FOOD

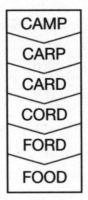

**NUMBER PYRAMID 1**

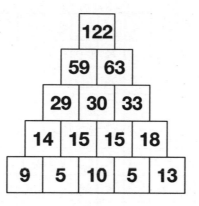

**NUMBER PYRAMID 2**

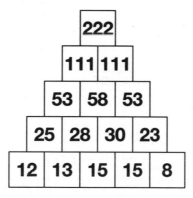

**BRAIN CHAIN 1**

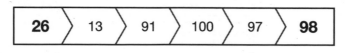

**BRAIN CHAIN 2**

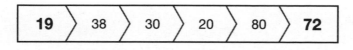

## NO FOUR IN A ROW 1

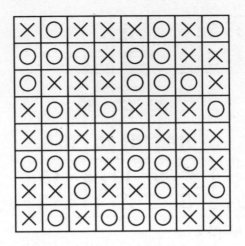

## NO FOUR IN A ROW 2

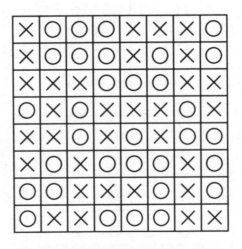

**DOMINOES 1**

| 3 | 6 | 6 | 1 | 5 | 2 | 1 | 3 |
|---|---|---|---|---|---|---|---|
| 5 | 5 | 2 | 3 | 0 | 6 | 1 | 3 |
| 1 | 2 | 5 | 4 | 4 | 1 | 4 | 4 |
| 6 | 6 | 3 | 0 | 0 | 3 | 0 | 0 |
| 3 | 4 | 5 | 5 | 4 | 6 | 2 | 6 |
| 0 | 1 | 5 | 0 | 1 | 6 | 2 | 1 |
| 0 | 2 | 5 | 2 | 2 | 4 | 4 | 3 |

**DOMINOES 2**

| 2 | 2 | 0 | 0 | 6 | 3 | 3 | 1 |
|---|---|---|---|---|---|---|---|
| 1 | 1 | 0 | 0 | 6 | 3 | 5 | 4 |
| 3 | 3 | 6 | 1 | 6 | 0 | 1 | 2 |
| 5 | 6 | 5 | 2 | 3 | 5 | 4 | 6 |
| 4 | 0 | 1 | 4 | 3 | 5 | 4 | 2 |
| 5 | 2 | 4 | 5 | 6 | 2 | 4 | 2 |
| 6 | 1 | 0 | 5 | 3 | 1 | 4 | 0 |

## CODE-BREAKING PUZZLES

### 1. Morse code

1. Defuse the IED
2. Launch a counter-attack
3. Your army needs you
4. Be the best
5. Critical terrain
6. Protect the nation

### 2. Semaphore

1. Realise your potential
2. Moral courage
3. Burst of fire

### Semaphore clock codes

1. Trust your team
2. Load the machine gun
3. Send back-up

### 3. Caesar shift

1. MEET EVERY CHALLENGE
2. CALL THE BOMB DISPOSAL TEAM
3. CALL THE MAJOR GENERAL (Shift: 4)
4. CONTACT, WAIT OUT (Shift: 2)
5. YOU'RE IN YOUR OWN TIME NOW (Shift: 23 – or backwards by 3)
6. IMPROVISED EXPLOSIVE DEVICE (Shift: 6)

### 4. Atbash

1. MILITARY OPERATIONS
2. I'M PROMOTING YOU TO LIEUTENANT
3. THIS PLATOON HAS THIRTY SOLDIERS

4. CONGRATULATIONS, LANCE CORPORAL
5. USE THE STREAM AS COVER
6. WE ARE UNDER ATTACK

## 5. Coded letters

**NATO codewords**
The NATO codewords are highlighted:

> Ms Caroline Scott
> 37 Pipe Road
> Mumbai
> India

Dear Mike,

*I was very glad to receive your letter, I'm happy you are doing well and progressing so quickly. It sounds like Charlie is getting up to plenty of mischief, as usual! He always was something of an alpha male.*

*Papa is the same as ever, he went to the shops for washing powder today and came back with three aubergines and a new bin for the bathroom. We are starting a tango class on Monday, which should be a fun challenge. The uniform is very strict, I have to buy some special dancing shoes with high heels – I have found a brand called Romeo which seems quite good value.*

*Do you have any holiday plans? We are thinking of going to Echo Point in the north of the country for a long weekend – not quite the same as our usual trip to the Ganges Delta, but it should make a pleasant change.*

*All my love,*
*Caroline*

So the hidden phrase is IMCAPTURED, or in other words: *I'M CAPTURED*.

## A punctual letter

Morse code has been used in the punctuation (as hinted at by 'punctual' in the title) to communicate the secret word RIFLES. The punctuation used in each paragraph, in order, gives you the code for one letter.

*Dear Major,*

*I am a Captain in the Royal Engineers posted in Brunei. I am writing to inform you of our progress on the training exercises we have been assigned – so far everything is going well.* Code: R .-.

*The troops are in good spirits and are supporting each other well. The only problem we have encountered is fatigue in the difficult conditions.* Code: I ..

*Exercises in the jungle naturally bring some challenges and some soldiers have been badly bitten by insects. Mosquitos in particular are proving a nuisance. We are running low on medication to treat these wounds – some more supplies would be greatly appreciated.* Code: F ..-.

*We have completed half of the training exercises and some of the new recruits show great promise. Particularly our latest addition from Sandhurst – Max. His ingenuity in the field is second to none.* Code: L .-..

*I hope all is going well in your regiment.* Code: E .

*I will be sending further updates once we have completed the remainder of the exercises. If you have any news about the supplies, please let myself and my medical team know. I look forward to hearing from you.* Code: S ...

*Regards,*
*Mark*

The resulting Morse code is:

.-. / .. / ..-. / .-.. / . / ...

So it reads: RIFLES.

## Letter code
The words 'dot' and 'dash' have been hidden variously in the letter to spell out, in Morse code, the word ENEMIES. Each paragraph contains the code for exactly one letter, as follows:

*Dear Dottie,*      CODE: dot = E
*It was wonderful to receive your last letter; it sounds like the cicadas have come out in full force! Your anecdotes always give us a good laugh.*      CODE: dash, dot = N

*We have just got back to base after a four-day-long training exercise and proper beds are proving a much-needed antidote.*      CODE: dot = E

*We haven't seen a great deal of wildlife while we have been out here, but yesterday that all changed very suddenly. A huge anaconda shot out of the undergrowth onto the path and we had to dash out of the way. Thankfully it seemed to have its eyes fixed on something to eat already.*      CODE: dash, dash = M

*Training is challenging as ever; our new sergeant likes to make sure we have dotted all our 'i's and crossed our 't's. I do tend to get up around an hour early to clean my kit and make sure everything is in order.*      CODE: dot, dot = I

*As part of our schedule, we have watched other regiments nearby doing their exercises – it's quite an experience seeing how other sergeants and new recruits operate.*      CODE: dot = E

*It would be lovely to organise a visit soon; I know we discussed a few dates but I have checked other times and there seems to be a good selection. We all have a lot to do this week, but hopefully after next Monday it won't be so much of a to-do to work something out.* CODE: dot, dot, dot = S

*All my love,*
*Jess*

So the Morse code is:

.../ -./ ./ --/ ../ ./ ...

And it reads: ENEMIES.

## 6. Numerical codes

These numbered codes use the 'A1Z26' system, where each letter of the alphabet is given a number from 1 to 26, A being 1 and Z being 26. The names of the first four barracks are:

1. Beachley
2. Raglan
3. Baker
4. Londesborough

The next two use the A1Z26 system in reverse, so that A is 26 and Z is 1. The number 0 represents a space.

5. Claro
6. Royal Artillery

In the final two codes, the original A1Z26 code is used, but the vowels are replaced as follows: A = 01, E = 02, I = 03, O = 04, U = 05 (with the '0' prefix as shown).

7. Bhurtpore
8. Redford

## 7. Anagram puzzles

### A unit of confusion
1. Brigade
2. Battlegroup
3. Battalion
4. Regiment
5. Company
6. Squadron
7. Platoon
8. Troop

The extras letters spell out the word *Division*.

### Unscramble the ranks
1. Brigadier
2. Captain
3. Colonel
4. Corporal
5. General
6. Lieutenant
7. Major
8. Private
9. Sergeant

10. Sergeant Major
11. Warrant Officer

*Officer Ranks:*
    Lieutenant
    Captain
    Major
    Colonel
    Brigadier
    General

*Soldier Ranks:*
    Private
    Corporal
    Sergeant
    Warrant Officer
    Sergeant Major

## Personal equipment

1. Gun
2. Radio
3. Grenade
4. Helmet
5. Body armour
6. Combat clothing

## ENIGMATIC PUZZLES

### 1. Army units

DIVISION
BRIGADE
BATTALION
REGIMENT
COMPANY
SQUADRON
PLATOON
TROOP

### 2. Officer ranks

BRI+GAD+IER (Brigadier)
CAP+TA+IN (Captain)
COL+ON+EL (Colonel)
GEN+ER+AL (General)
LIE+UTE+NA+NT (Lieutenant)
MA+JOR (Major)

### 3. British beasts

You may have A and B the other way around to the table below, but the solution is as follows:

| Rule A | Rule B | Rules A + B | Neither A nor B |
|--------|--------|-------------|-----------------|
| Challenger | Cook | Churchill | Cleaner |
| Centurion | Chaplin | Cromwell | Car |

Rule A: Names of British tanks
Rule B: Surnames of notable British historical figures

## 4. An unusual occupation

Army Nurse
Bricklayer
Dog Handler
Driver
Guardsman
Mariner
Musician
Officer
Paratrooper

## 5. African deployments

South Sudan
Somalia
Democratic Republic of the Congo
Kenya
Nigeria
Gabon
Malawi

## 6. A start in the army

| | |
|---|---|
| Avant-garde | Novel and experimental |
| Balls to the wall | Complete a task with intense effort |
| Bite the bullet | Deal with the inevitable displeasure |
| Loose cannon | An unpredictable character |
| No man's land | Unclaimed territory |
| On the double | Very quickly |
| Take the flak | Endure strong criticism |

### 7. Ancient civilisations

- Trojan
- Titan
- Juno
- Spartan

These are all types of British military vehicle. The Spartan is for reconnaissance, the Titan is a bridge launcher, the Juno is a helicopter and the Trojan is an armoured engineer vehicle.

## MEMORY TESTS

### 5. Sleep test

**Questions**
1. Seven to eight hours
2. One hour
3. Three
4. Nine
5. Consuming caffeine or alcohol

### 6. Follow the difference

*When you reach the footpath, cross directly over the stream and continue north at a steady rate. In 30 km you'll reach a sharp incline with a bridleway in front of you. Cross the bridleway (remember to look out for horses!) and follow the footpath up the steep hill. Be careful – once you reach the top there's a steep drop on the eastern side. Nice spot for a picnic! Sun will rise at around 2000 hrs on Wednesday, so as long as you've got great visibility, you'll have plenty of time left when the hike is over. Remember to open the gates behind you.*

### 8. Kit bag

The compass is missing.

## 10. Grid memory

The image is a tick, confirming that you solved the puzzle correctly.

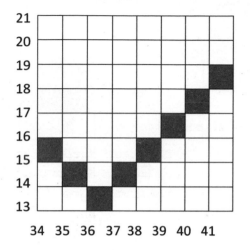

## 11. Fit as a fiddle

Questions
1. Thirty sit-ups
2. Forty-five in total
3. Squats
4. Fifteen minutes
5. Six stages – with press-ups repeated

## 13. Names and numbers

Questions
1. 2 x 3 = 6
2. 2 + 1 = 3
3. 6 – 4 = 2
4. 8 – 8 = 0
5. 1 + 1 + 2 + 2 = George (6)

For the bonus: these names all belong to kings and queens of England, and the numbers tell you how many monarchs have ruled with that name.

### 14. Memory maths

1.

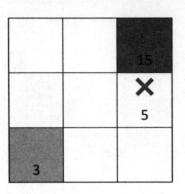

$15 \div 3 = 5$

2.

$9 \times 4 = 36$

**3.**

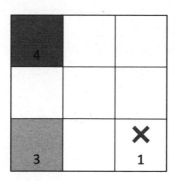

$4 - 3 = 1$

**4.**

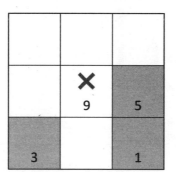

$5 + 3 + 1 = 9$

## 15. Word association

### Questions
1. Orange
2. Boots; the goggles were above, and the map to the left
3. Truck
4. Banana – it's paired with the helicopter

## 17. Remember this recipe

**Questions**

1. Three – carrots, onions and red peppers
2. Two kilograms
3. Red peppers
4. Ten
5. Sausages
6. Ten minutes

## 18. Reconnaissance ready

You should exit through the east gate. Sentry points are marked with a dot.

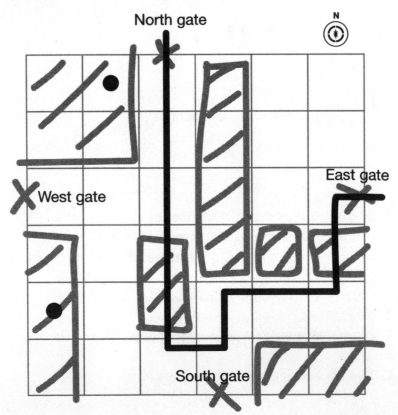

# KNOWLEDGE TESTS

### 1. British Army quiz

1. a. Chief of the General Staff (CGS). As of 2019, the incumbent CGS is General Sir Mark Carleton-Smith
2. c. General (also known as a four-star general)
3. b. Bolivia
4. b. Army Officer Selection Board
5. c. 7 – They are: Private, Lance Corporal, Corporal, Sergeant, Staff/Colour Sergeant, Warrant Officer Class 2, Warrant Officer Class 1
6. a. Multi-terrain pattern (MTP)
7. a. Andover

### 2. History of the British Army quiz

1. c. 1947
2. b. Falklands War
3. b. 1960
4. a. The union of England and Scotland

### 3. British monarchy quiz

1. b. Prince Harry
2. a. Queen Elizabeth II
3. c. Samoa. Although it is a member of the Commonwealth of Nations, Samoa does not have Elizabeth II as its monarch. It is therefore not one of the 16 Commonwealth Realms
4. b. The 1st Buckingham Palace Company was a Girl Guide patrol, created so that Princess Elizabeth (now Elizabeth II) could become a Girl Guide

### 4. UK geography quiz

1. a. Ben Nevis. Scafell Pike is the highest mountain in England, and Snowdon the highest in Wales
2. c. River Severn, which runs through England and Wales
3. c. 48
4. b. 15
5. c. 20 per cent. According to National Parks, 19.9 per cent of Wales is designated National Park – more than the combined percentages in Scotland and England
6. a. Skaw, Unst. Part of the Shetland Isles, Unst is the northernmost inhabited island in the UK, and Skaw is its northernmost settlement
7. a. Berkshire
8. b. Derbyshire. It is 113 kilometres from the nearest coast in any direction
9. c. The River Tees. The waterfall is located in County Durham
10. b. 4 – England, Wales, Scotland and Northern Ireland

If you are interested in exploring further the role of the British Army and possible careers, please scan the QR code below or visit www.army.mod.uk